I0039437

The Authorities

Powerful Wisdom from Leaders in the Field

RALSTON POWELL

Simple Steps for Big Results in Boosting Heart Health

AuthoritiesPress

ISBN: 978-1-77277-149-7

Publisher
Authorities Press
Markham, ON
Canada

Printed in Canada and the United States of America

FOREWORD

Experts are to be admired for their knowledge, but they often remain unrecognized by the general public because they save their information and insights for paying customers and clients. There are many experts in a given field, but their impact is limited to the handful of people with whom they work.

Unlike experts, authorities share their knowledge and expertise far more broadly, so they make a big impact on the world. Authorities become known and admired as leading experts and, as such, typically do very well economically and professionally. Most authorities are also mature enough to know that part of the joy of monetary success is the accompanying moral and spiritual obligation to give back.

Many people want to learn and work with well-respected and generous authorities, but don't always know where to find them. They may be known to their peers, or within a specific community, but have not had the opportunity to reach a wider audience. At one time, they might have submitted a proposal to the For Dummies or Chicken Soup for the Soul series of books, but it's now almost impossible to get accepted as a new author in such branded book series.

It is more than fitting that Raymond Aaron, an internationally known and respected authority in his own right, would be the one to recognize the need for a new venue in which authorities could share their considerable knowledge with readers everywhere. As the only author ever to be included in both of the book series mentioned above, Raymond has had the opportunity to give back and he understands how crucial it is for authorities to have a platform from which to share their expertise.

I have known and worked with Raymond for a number of years and consider him a valued friend and talented coach. He knows how to spot talented and knowledgeable people and he desires to see them prosper. Over the years, success coaching and speaking engagements around the world have made it possible for Raymond to meet many of these talented authorities. He recognizes and relates to their passion and enthusiasm for what they do, as well as their desire to share what they know. He tells me that's why he created this new nonfiction branded book series, *The Authorities*.

Dr. Nido Qubein
President, High Point University

TABLE OF CONTENTS

ADVANCED PRAISE FOR RALSTON POWELL

I have known Ralston Powell for over 16 years. I would describe him as a very kind, generous and loving man. Ralston is a God-fearing person who proudly shares his religious beliefs with others. Ralston always presents a very warm, caring and gentle personality, quite evident in the way in which he cares for me. Every Sunday Ralston drives me to Church. When he picks me up, he gently assists me to the car and extends the same courtesy on our return home. Ralston is extremely generous with his time. During the summer, he is always available to assist me with my vegetable and flower gardens. He surely has a green thumb.

Ralston has become a big part of my family and is loved by all. He partakes in our family Christmas, Thanksgiving and Sunday dinners. We always welcome his presence. Ralston, I cannot thank you enough for being a big part of my life and my family. You have always been an inspiration and a blessing to us!

Ralston, I dedicate this Scripture reading to you:

"My son, attend to my words; incline thine ear unto my sayings. Let them not depart from thine eyes; keep them in the midst of thine heart. For they are life unto those that find them, and health to all their flesh. Keep thy heart with all diligence; for out of it are the issues of life." Proverbs 4:20-23

— Catherine Charles
Richmond Hill, Ontario

We first met Ralston at an event gathering about eight years ago in Toronto. He is a quiet, kind and approachable man. We quickly learned Ralston is not just an ordinary guy. He emits love, patience and kindness to everyone he encounters. His faithfulness, dedication and persistence are inspirational. It is further undergirded by a lifestyle, which took us by surprise. Whenever we see Ralston he has a welcoming smile on his face and an outstretched hand to shake or hug to give. This in itself is a rare quality to possess; yet after years of knowing him we have found that he gets up very early in the morning, works long grueling hours, driving through several cities, and still radiates love and warmth to whomever he encounters. He constantly sacrifices his time, going out of his way to help others in anyway he can! Given the same situation, many of us would look at the hardships and challenges of life and make excuses; saying we are too tired, too busy or that we do not have the appropriate resources. When we look at Ralston, we see a man with a positive, healthy mindset and attitude allowing him to break down walls between himself and others. This mindset is one of Ralston's greatest attributes for possessing and maintaining a healthy, fulfilling, and meaningful life. As we have grown in our friendship, we cherish and listen to the wisdom of not only Ralston's words, but his lifestyle as well. We encourage you now, as a reader, to look deep into the wisdom presented in his book. It will enhance your life. How do we know? We know from experience, Ralston has touched our lives and that of many other lives surrounding him for the better!

— Andrew Jones, Youth Leadership
& Azeb Jones, Song Leader
Whitby, Ontario

It is my blessing to be asked by Mr. Ralston Powell, a man who trusts his spiritual and physical health in our Almighty God, to write my opinion about his recent publication in regards to heart health.

Mr. Powell lays out a clear road map to recovery for the millions of people needlessly suffering from heart disease. He provides you with recommendations for changes in diets, supplements and environment to assist people dealing with, and even reversing, heart conditions.

Mr. Powell gives you both the knowledge and solutions to heart health. You just need to apply them.

— Dr. Francis K. Long, Dentist
Richmond Hill, Ontario

INTRODUCTION

This book introduces you to *The Authorities* — individuals who have distinguished themselves in life and in business. Authorities make a big impact on the world. Authorities are leaders in their chosen fields. Authorities typically do very well financially, and are evolved enough to know that part of the joy of monetary success is the accompanying social, moral and spiritual obligation to give back.

Authorities are not just outstanding. They are also *known* to be outstanding.

This additional element begins to explain the difference between two strategic business and life concepts — one that seems great, but isn't, and the other that fills in the essential missing gap of the first.

The first concept is "the expert."

What is an expert? The real definition is …

EXPERT: *a person who knows stuff*

People who have attained a very senior academic degree (like a PhD or an MD) definitely know stuff. People who read voraciously and retain what they read definitely know stuff. Unfortunately, just because you know stuff does not mean that anyone respects the fact that you do. Even though some experts are successful, alas, most are not — because knowing stuff is not enough.

Well, then, what is the missing piece?

What the expert lacks, "the authority" has. The authority both knows stuff and is *known* to know stuff. So, more simply …

AUTHORITY: *a person who is known as an expert*

The difference is not subtle. The difference is not merely semantic. The difference is enormous.

When it comes to this subject, there are actually three categories in which people fall:

- People who don't know much and are unsuccessful in life and in business. Most people fall in this category.
- People who know stuff, but still don't leave much of a footprint in the world. There are a lot of people like this.
- Experts who are also ***known*** as experts become authorities and authorities are always wondrously successful. Authorities are able to contribute more to humanity through both their chosen work and their giving back.

This book is about the highest category, *The Authorities* — people who have reached the peak in their field and are known as such.

You will definitely know some of *The Authorities* in this book, especially since there are some world-famous ones. Others are just as exceptional, but you may not yet know about them. Our featured author, for example, is Ralston Powell. A man of tremendous faith, Ralston began life on the island of Jamaica. He attended Linstead Primary, St. Georges Preparatory, and Dintahill Tech. Trainings Centre where he studied English, Math, and Chemistry. His first job was with P.E. Stanigar and Sons, where he was a sales and billing clerk.

After immigrating to Canada as a young man, he continued the same lifestyle and furthered his education. He attended Broncondale Gospel Hall and then went to The Prayer Palace with Pastor Paul, Cathy, Tim and Tom. He also attended the church called Kabod Ministries with Angela Grant, before attending Koinonia Worship Center which is now called The Access Center with Dr. Daniel Sichelhi.

A dramatic change came into his life when he started to work at the airport with airport special delivery service. He then worked with Cottrell Air, Fast Air, and now currently works with Ceva Freight.

Ralston had the joy of going to Israel and walking the place where Jesus walked. It was one of the most fulfilling experiences of his life.

He was privileged to go to California and meet with Real Estate icon Robert Allen, where he had a one-on-one dialogue with him.

Ralston became so concerned about how heart disease is becoming more prevalent and widespread even in healthy, young people that he felt compelled to educate himself on the problem. In *The Authorities*, Ralston provides tips for cutting down your own chances of getting heart disease. Read Ralston's chapter, "Simple Steps for Big Results in Boosting Heart Health," where he shares his knowledge on a heart-healthy lifestyle. With his guidance, you will discover major risk factors and manageable steps you can take to improve your heart health.

To be considered for inclusion in a subsequent edition of *The Authorities*, register to attend a future event at www.aaron.com/events where you will be interviewed and considered.

Simple Steps for Big Results in Boosting Heart Health

RALSTON POWELL

"First say to yourself what you would be: and then do what you have to do."
— Epictetus

It strikes like lightning, and it steals loved ones from their families. It is the number one killer of men and women in Western societies; twelve million people die from it each year around the world. While some of its warning signs are obvious, it can come disguised as flu, headache, or just plain fatigue.

Some people have no symptoms and do not see it coming. They are oblivious to the damage that is already done until they are at severe risk of a catastrophe. It can happen at any time, even when they are at rest. If you do not act fast enough or seek help within minutes, it can be fatal.

What am I talking about here? What is this disease that takes lives by stealth, which can recur even when you've recovered from it?

A heart attack.

How many of you have lost a loved one, a friend, or a colleague to a heart attack? Sadly enough, there are many of us in these ranks. It is clear that people are getting sick and dying even at a young age. In fact, I first became concerned about the rising incidence of both heart disease and cancer when a member of my church died of Leukemia. This man was young, approximately 30 years old with a wife and young children. At the time, anyone who was diagnosed with cancer of the blood felt a sense of hopelessness. The second time I felt a sense of concern was when I heard of the death of a young man at a prominent company that I would visit daily. His diagnosis was a massive heart attack. Following that, a friend and co-worker who was having problems with his heart went on vacation to Guyana; in the heat, he suffered a massive heart attack and died. These experiences made me concerned enough to do research, and I found out that heart disease is stated to be North America's number one killer. People from all walks of life can be affected.

Heart disease is commonly reported among those who are physically unfit, carry too much weight, who smoke and drink heavily, and who are eating fat-rich foods. Yet it is no longer just the plight of middle-aged men. Women are just as susceptible, especially after menopause.

Tragically, there are now stories that heart disease is striking the seemingly healthy. You can be a marathon runner, observe a low-calorie diet, have manageable cholesterol, and you can still suffer a catastrophic heart attack without any notice or warning signs.

WHAT IS A HEART ATTACK?

Your heart is no bigger than a fist, but it is your strongest organ, and it works tirelessly from the time you take your first breath to your last. It is made of cardiac muscle, a specialized muscle that only exists in the heart, and, unlike muscles in our legs or arms, the cardiac muscle never tires.

The heart works to pump life-giving oxygen and nutrients in the blood to every part of your body. On average, it beats between 60-100 times per minute at rest. When you work out or are feeling anxious or angry, your heart beats more quickly.

Feeding the heart with blood are the coronary arteries. When there is too much cholesterol in the bloodstream, it gets deposited on the inner linings of these blood vessels, just like rust on the insides of old plumbing. These deposits, called plaque, build up and block oxygen from getting to the heart.

Decreased blood flow causes chest pain, angina, or shortness of breath. A complete blockage of blood flow can damage or destroy part of the heart muscle. Typical symptoms of an attack are anxiety, sweating, chest pain, stiffness or discomfort in the upper body, nausea, and stomach pain.

A person can survive a heart attack due, in part, to significant improvements in medical treatment, yet the statistics are ugly. More than 60% of people who suffer a heart attack die before getting the medical help that they need.

WHAT'S THE GOOD NEWS HERE?

The good news is that a heart attack is absolutely preventable. And its damage is reversible. If you've suffered the disease before, you can empower yourself to make sure you'll never be victim to another attack again. You can do so with minimal or zero drug use or surgical interventions, such as a coronary bypass or having stents placed in your arteries to improve blood flow.

You can lead a healthier life by making easy lifestyle changes. These adjustments are so simple you can see results within a month. Not only that, but you also reduce the risks against you by more than half.

Pretty good news, isn't it?

Changing the way you live is far more effective in prevention and repair than any number of drugs or tubes put into your body. Treating only the symptoms or the risks is taking the short-view, and that is why, once your doctor prescribes medication, you are on it for the rest of your life. You can stop playing the victim and take back control of your own life. By investing some time and committing to making the changes, you can protect yourself from this devastating disease and live life fully.

HEALTH IS OUR BIRTHRIGHT

It is time for a paradigm shift in the way we look at the prevention of heart disease and its therapy for rehabilitation. We must go beyond the conventional attitudes and treatments that limit how we can live healthier lives.

The first step we must take is to change the way we look at our health. I've always firmly believed that health is our birthright. Our bodies are wonderful, complex, finely-tuned instruments. There're no two ways of saying it - it is a miracle!

Picture this. You make a small cut on your finger when you're cutting vegetables. You may run tap water over the finger to stop the bleeding, pour hydrogen peroxide on it, and apply a band-aid. Since it was a small and superficial cut, you're completely healed within a few days. Voila!

But what has taken place without conscious intervention from you is a sequence of healing events. The moment the skin is cut, the blood vessels feeding blood to the area miraculously reduce blood flow to the injured area, like turning off the tap. Next, platelets rush to the scene. They have been alerted to the emergency by enzymes released from the damaged blood vessels. The platelets clot together to form a plug that becomes a scab to stop the blood vessel from bleeding further. In the meantime, signals are sent out to more platelets to come help at the site of the damage.

When the bleeding is under control, the constricted blood vessels open up again, this time bringing important white blood cells to destroy any germs or infections that may have gotten into the body through the wound. Then the body concentrates on healing and rebuilding. The skin on both sides of the cut stretches to meet in the middle, forming a scar, which may or may not disappear as the body adds more collagen to the area. The finger is almost as good as new.

Notice that I said all of this happened without any conscious thought on your part. That's because you are gifted with a terrific immune system with enormous healing power, which orchestrates events to repair and renew your body even as you're reading this sentence.

TIME TO GET SMART ABOUT HEART HEALTH

Why does disease happen then? When we are out of balance, both physically and emotionally, we suppress our immune functions. We turn our body from its natural alkaline state in which disease cannot flourish to an acidic state, which is ripe ground for illnesses like heart diseases and diabetes.

We need to look at health as being much more than just being free of disease. We should look at health as the perfect mind-body balance and the platform from which we can reach our highest potential, our greatest creativity, and lasting happiness.

At this point, I wish to reiterate that power lies within you.

What if there is a history of heart disease in your family? Doesn't it run in the genes? It is mistaken thinking to blame it on a shared heritage. Heart attacks are caused by how the environment affects your genes. So, really, it is what you eat, how much or little you exercise, how you handle stress, and environmental toxins that cause hypertension, high cholesterol, and other imbalances such as high blood sugar that increase the risk of a heart attack.

By turning from victim to someone who takes control with courage and determination, you will make healthy choices, add beneficial foods, exercises, therapies, and natural supplements to your lifestyle. Remember to be kind to yourself and take baby steps, but also congratulate yourself for every accomplishment, no matter how small.

CUT BACK RISK FACTORS

The number of things that make us more vulnerable to heart attacks are called risk factors. Research shows that poor lifestyle choices heighten some of these risk factors, including:

- Smoking

- o Unhealthy diet
- o Insufficient exercise
- o Chronic stress

These unfortunate lifestyle decisions lead to physical problems such as high blood pressure, high blood sugar, and a high level of blood fats. High blood pressure forces the heart to work harder than it should, causing it to weaken faster over time. High blood sugar speeds up the narrowing and the hardening of the arteries. We have already discussed the damage to the heart from high cholesterol levels.

Unrelieved stress from feeling anxious, lonely, isolated, or angry also causes significant damage. It is hard to accept that stress can be the single trigger for a heart attack. But stress creates that string of events that can lead to that one, catastrophic heart attack. Stress raises cholesterol levels, aggravates blood sugar imbalances, and elevates blood pressure, all of which make the blood more likely to clot.

In plain speak, the more risk factors there are in your life, the higher the risk you run of a heart attack.

SIMPLE STEPS, BIG RESULTS

There are steps you can take, starting now. It is better for you to add one simple change every day rather than attempt to do everything at once and give up down the road because you're overwhelmed by having to do too much at any one time.

Here are a few suggestions of what you can do:

1. Stop smoking. You reduce the odds of a heart attack from the very

moment you stop using tobacco.

2. Move it, move it, move it. Medical literature recommends exercising 30 minutes or more several days of the week. But in a pinch, even ten minutes of intense physical exercise goes a long way to making a difference. Take the stairs rather than the escalator, take a walk during lunch, get off at an earlier stop and walk the last few blocks to work or home.

3. Eat heart-healthy foods. Five servings of fruit and vegetables are a daily must, and if you must snack, pick vegetables like carrots, cucumbers, peppers, or fruit. Avoid the temptation to indulge in a sugar-rich pastry. Other heart-healthy foods are lean meats, fish, low-fat dairy, and beans.

4. Load up on antioxidants. These are the nutrients that repair daily damage to your arteries. Fruits and vegetables contain antioxidants. Green tea is another source of antioxidants; it has several powerful antioxidants that reduce cholesterol levels.

5. Cut back on fats. Reduce trans fats from margarine and avoid saturated fats, which are fats that turn solid at room temperature such as butter, cheese, and animal fats. Use olive oil as a substitute for butter or margarine and make sure you buy cold-pressed extra virgin oil as it has more of the healthy antioxidants.

6. Support with supplements. Pick antioxidant vitamin supplements such as Vitamin E and B vitamins, including B6 and folic acid. Add healthy omega-3 fats to your diet by sprinkling a couple of tablespoons of pre-ground flaxseed to your salad, smoothies, or cereal. Flaxseed oil, like fish oil, has been shown in studies to reduce certain cardiac risk factors.

7. Get regular check-ups. Consult with your doctor, but also broaden your choices by seeking advice from natural therapy providers such as

a naturopath or nutritionist. No one knows it all, and you must take responsibility for your own health. Conduct research and catch up on the latest reading.

8. Get good quality sleep. When we sleep, we give the body time and space to carry out the repair work to heal and to boost good health. Insufficient sleep is linked to weight gain, high blood pressure, and other heart disease risk factors. Sufficient sleep is defined as between seven to nine hours.

BOOST HEALING BY CREATING A HEALING ENVIRONMENT

Reducing stress is a major ingredient in the recipe for good health, so find ways to relieve stress in your life. Rethink a tendency to overwork in the office and sort out your priorities so you do not get too upset when work is frustrating. Build support groups and nurture strong relationships. Emotional support from friends and family are stress buffers.

Stack up on stress management tools. There are so many relaxation techniques available to any of us, such as yoga, Tai Chi, Qigong, acupuncture, or guided meditations. Yoga has become commonplace with many community centers offering classes. Acupuncture is recommended as a natural remedy to rebalance the body's energy flow, improve circulation, and blood flow to the heart.

Meditation has been shown to lower cholesterol and reverse any thickening of the carotid arteries. You can join meditation groups, download soothing music, and even find free guided meditations online which you can follow within the sanctuary of your own home. The idea is to have fun and experiment to see which one resonates best with you. Be committed and consistent with the relaxation techniques of your choice; you are making great strides towards better health.

Here's another tip: Do you know how health and beauty spas get you to slow down and chill out by playing slow, meditative music? Notice that they do not have loud rock-and-roll because meditative melodies slow the heart rate, while loud and fast beats rev up our natural heart rate. Prepare a playlist of soft, soothing music to help you take it down a notch.

PAY HEED TO THE MIND-BODY CONNECTION

Health is not just a state of the body, it is also a state of mind. Our bodies react to what we think and how we feel, and the mind-body connection is constantly in play.

It shouldn't surprise you that one of the best mind-body exercises is to have a good laugh. Laughter is the best medicine. We've all heard this before, and it is such a common saying that we often overlook how true the advice is. When you laugh out loud, you can't stay depressed, angry, or frustrated. In fact, a good belly laugh turns these negative emotions on their head.

When you're laughing until your sides hurt, you're doing many good things for your body: You're giving the T-cells a good boost. These are special white blood cells that are crucial to the immune system. They regulate the immune response or directly swoop down on infected cells. The T-cells need to be activated, and a good laugh will do precisely that.

Laughing promotes a sense of well-being. Endorphins are the feel-good chemicals that are produced from exercise. Laughter produces a healthy dose of endorphins and also contributes to an overall positive outlook on life. Those who have a more positive attitude tend to stay healthier or recover faster.

Your body relaxes for up to 45 minutes after laughing. Furthermore, laughter is contagious. Sharing a laugh with someone lowers barriers, promotes intimacy, and enhances relationships, all of which are good things that boost heart health.

Set your mind towards optimal health and successful healing. The change in attitude may seem like a small step, but before you know it, you've made giant strides towards maintaining a healthy heart.

Branding Small Business

RAYMOND AARON

Branding is an incredibly important tool for creating and building your business. Large companies have been benefiting from branding ever since people first started selling things to other people. Branding made those businesses big.

If you're a small business owner, you probably imagine that small companies are different and don't need branding as much as large companies do. Not true. The truth is small businesses need branding just as much, if not more, than large companies.

Perhaps you've thought about branding, but assumed you'd need millions of dollars to do it properly, or that branding is just the same thing as marketing. Nothing could be further from the truth.

Marketing is the engine of your company's success. Branding is the fuel in that engine.

In the old days, salespeople were a big part of the selling process. They recommended one product over another and laid out the reasons why it was better. Salespeople had credibility because they knew about all the products, and customers often took the advice they had to offer.

Today, consumers control the buying process. They shop in big box stores, super-sized supermarkets, and over the Internet — where there are no salespeople. Buyers now get online and gather information beforehand. They learn about all the products available and look to see if there really is any difference between them. Consumers also read reviews and check social media to see if both the company and the product are reputable. In other words, they want to know what the brand is all about.

The way of commerce used to be: "Nothing happens till something is sold." Today it's: "Nothing happens till something is branded!"

DEFINING A BRAND

A brand is a proper name that stands for something. It lives in the consumer's mind, has positive or negative characteristics, and invokes a feeling or an image. In short, it's a person's perception of a product or a company.

When all goes well, consumers associate the same characteristics with a brand that the company talks about in its advertising, public relations, marketing and sales materials. Of course, when a product doesn't live up to what the company says about it, the brand gets a bad reputation. On the other hand, if a product or service over-delivers on the promises made, the brand can become a superstar.

RECOGNIZING BRANDING AND ITS CHARACTERISTICS

Branding is the science and art of making something that isn't unique, unique. Branding in the marketplace is the same as branding on a ranch. On a ranch, ranchers use branding to differentiate their cattle from every other rancher's cattle (because all cattle look pretty much the same). In the marketplace, branding is what makes a product stand out in a crowd of similar products. The right branding gets you noticed, remembered and sold — or perhaps I should say bought, because today it is all about buying, not selling.

There are four main characteristics of branding that make it an integral part of the marketing and purchasing process.

1. Branding makes you trustworthy and known

Branding makes a product more special than other products. With branding, a normal, everyday product has a personality, and a first and last name, and people know who you are.

In today's marketplace, most products are, more or less, just like their competition. Toilet paper is toilet paper, milk is milk, and a grocery store by any other name is still a grocery store. However, branding takes a product and makes it unique. For example, high-quality drinking water is available from just about every tap in the Western world and it's free, but people pay good money for it when it comes in a bottle. Branding takes bottled water and makes Evian.

Furthermore, every aspect of your brand gives potential customers a feeling or comfort level that they associate with you. The more powerful and positive that feeling is, the more easily and more frequently they will want to do business with you and, indeed, will do business with you.

2. Branding differentiates you from others

Strong branding makes you better than your competition, and makes your product name memorable and easy to remember. Even if your product is absolutely the same as every other product like it, branding makes it special. Branding makes it the first product a consumer thinks about when deciding to make a purchase.

Branding also makes a product seem popular. Everyone knows about it, which implicitly says people like it. And, if people like it, it must be good.

3. Branding makes you worth more money

The stronger your branding is, the more likely people are willing to spend that little bit extra because they believe you, your product, your service, or your business are worth it. They may say they won't, but they will. They do it all the time.

For example, a one-pound box of Godiva chocolates costs about $40; the same weight of Hershey's Kisses costs about $4. The quality of the chocolate isn't ten times greater. The reason people buy Godiva is that the brand Godiva means "gift" whereas the brand Hershey means "snack". Gifts obviously cost more than snacks.

4. Branding pre-sells your product

In the buying age, people most often make the decision on which products to pick up before they walk into the store. The stronger the branding, the more likely people are to think in terms of your product rather than the product category. For example, people are as likely, maybe even more likely, to add Hellmann's to the shopping list as they are to write down simply mayo. The same is true for soda, ketchup, and many other products with successful, strong branding.

Plus, as soon as a shopper gets to the shelf, branding can provide a quick reminder of what products to grab in a few ways:

- An icon or logo
- A specific color
- An audio icon

BRANDING IN A SMALL BUSINESS

Big companies spend millions of dollars on advertising, marketing, and public relations (PR) to build recognition of a new product name. They get their selling messages out to the public using television, radio, magazines, and the Internet. They can even throw money at damage control when necessary. The strategies for branding are the same in a small business, but the scale, costs, and a few of the tactics change.

Make your brand name work harder

The name of a small business can mean everything in terms of branding. Your brand name needs to work harder for your business than you do. It's the first thing a prospective customer sees, and it is how they will remember you. A brand name has to be memorable when spoken, and focused in its meaning. If the name doesn't represent what consumers believe about a product and the company that makes it, then that brand will fail.

In building your product's reputation and image, less is often significantly more. Make sure the name you choose immediately gives a sense of what you do.

Large corporations have millions of dollars to take a meaningless brand name and make it stand for something. Small businesses don't, so use words that really mean something. Strive for something interesting and be right on point. You don't need to be boring.

Plumbers, for example, would do well setting themselves apart with names like "The On-Time Plumber" or "24/7 Plumbing". The same is true for electricians, IT providers, or even marketing consultants. Plenty of other types of business are so general in nature they just don't work hard enough in a business or product name.

Even the playing field: The Net

The Internet has leveled the playing field for small businesses like nothing else. You can use the Internet in several ways to market your brand:

Website: Developing and maintaining a website is easier than ever. Anyone can find your business regardless of its size.

Social Media: Facebook and Twitter can promote your brand in a cost-effective manner.

BUILDING YOUR BRAND WITH THE BRANDING LADDER

Even if you do everything perfectly the first time (and I don't know anyone who does), branding takes time. How much time isn't just up to you, but you can speed things along by understanding the different levels of branding, as well as the business and marketing strategies that can get you to the top.

Introducing the Branding Ladder

Moving through the levels of branding is like climbing a ladder to the top of the marketplace. The Branding Ladder has five distinct rungs and, unlike stairs, you can't take them two at a time. You have to take them in order, and some businesses spend more time on each rung than others.

You can also think of the Branding Ladder in terms of a scale from zero to ten. Everyone starts at zero. If you properly climb the ladder, you can end up at 12 out of 10. The Branding Ladder below shows a special rung at the top of the ladder that can take your business over the top. The following section explains the Branding Ladder and how your small business can move up it.

THE BRANDING LADDER	
Brand Advocacy	**12/10**
Brand Insistence	**10/10**
Brand Preference	**3/10**
Brand Awareness	**1/10**
Brand Absence	**0/10**

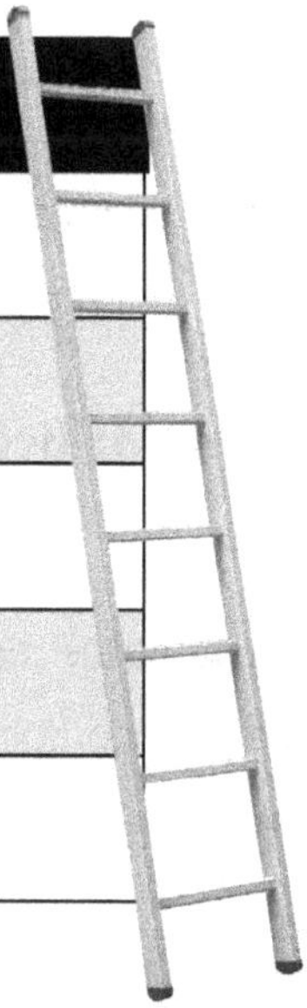

Rung 1: Living in the void

Your business, in fact every business, starts at the bottom rung, which is called brand absence, meaning you have no brand whatsoever except your own name. On a scale of one to ten, brand absence is, of course, zero. That's the worst place to live and obviously the most difficult entrepreneurially. The good news is that the only way is up.

Ninety-seven percent of businesses live on this rung of the Branding Ladder. They earn far less than they want to earn, far less than they should earn, and far less than they would earn if they did exactly the same work under a real brand.

Rung 2: Achieving awareness

Brand awareness is a good first step up the ladder to the second rung. Actually, it's really good, especially because 97 percent of businesses never get there. You want people to be aware of you. When person A speaks to person B and says, "Have you heard of "The 24/7 Plumber?" You want the answer to be "yes".

On that scale of one to ten, however, brand awareness is only a one. It's better than nothing, but not that much better. Although people know of your brand, being aware doesn't mean that they are interested in buying it. Coca Cola drinkers know about Pepsi, but they don't drink it.

Rung 3: Becoming the preferred brand

Getting to the third rung, brand preference, is definitely a real step up. This rung means that people prefer to use your product or service rather than that of your competition. They believe there is a real difference between you and others, and you're their first choice. This rung is a crucial branding stage for parity products, such as bottled water and breakfast cereals, not to mention plumbers, electricians, lawyers, and all the others. Brand preference is clearly better than brand awareness, but it's less than halfway up the ladder.

Car rental companies represent a perfect example of why brand preference may not be enough. When someone lands at an airport and needs to rent a car on the spot, he or she may go straight to the preferred rental counter. If that company has a car available, it's a sale. However, if all the cars for that company have been rented, the person will move to the next rental kiosk without much thought, because one rental car is just as good as another.

Exerting Brand Preference needs to be easy and convenient

If all you have is brand preference, your business is on shaky ground and you can lose business for the feeblest of reasons. Very few people go to a second or third supermarket just to find their favorite brand of bottled water. Similarly, a shopper may prefer one store over another but, if both stores sell the same products, he or she will often go to the closest store even if it is not the better liked one. The reason for staying nearby does not need to be a dramatic one — the shopper may simply be tired, on a tight schedule, or not in the mood to travel.

Rung 4: Making it you and only you

When your customers are so committed to your product or service that they won't accept a substitute, you have reached the fourth rung of the Branding Ladder. All companies strive to reach this place, called brand insistence.

Brand insistence means that someone's experience with a product in terms of performance, durability, customer service, and image has been sufficiently exceptional. As a result, the product has earned an incredible level of loyalty.

If the product isn't available where the customer is, he or she will literally not buy something else. Rather, the person will look for the preferred product elsewhere. Can you imagine what a fabulous place this is for a company to be? Brand insistence is the best of the best, the perfect ten out of ten, the whole ball of wax.

Apple is a perfect example of brand insistence

Apple users don't just think, they know in their heads and hearts, that anything made by Apple is technologically-advanced, user-friendly, and just all-around superior. Committed to everything Apple, Mac users won't even entertain the thought that a PC may have positive attributes.

Apple people love everything about their Macs, iPads, iPhones, the Mac stores and all those apps. When the company introduces a new product, many of its brand-insistent fans actually wait in line overnight to be one of the first to have it. Steve Jobs is one of their idols.

Considering one big potential problem

Unfortunately, you can lose brand insistence much more quickly than you can achieve it. Brand-insistent customers have such high expectations that they can be disillusioned or disappointed by just one bad product experience. You also have to consistently reinforce the positives because insistence can fade over time. Even someone who has bought and re-bought a specific brand of car for the last 20 years can decide it's just time for a change. That's how fickle the world is.

At ten out of ten, brand insistence may seem like the top rung of the ladder, but it's not. One rung is actually better, and it involves getting your brand-insistent customers to keep polishing your brand for you.

Rung 5: Getting customers to do the work for you

Brand advocacy is the highest rung on the ladder. It's better than ten out of ten because you have customers who are so happy with your product that they want everyone to know about it and use it. Think of them as uber-fans. Not only do they recommend you to friends and family, they also practically shout your praises from the rooftops, interrupt conversations among strangers to give their opinion, and tell everyone they meet how fantastic you are. Most companies can only aspire to this level of customer satisfaction. Apple is one of the few large corporations in recent history that has brand advocates all over the world.

- Brand advocacy does the following five extraordinary things for your company. Brand advocacy:

- Provides a level of visibility that you couldn't pay for if you tried. Brand advocates are so enthusiastic they talk about you all the time, and reach people in ways general media and public relations can't. You get great visibility because they make sure people actually listen.

- Delivers free advertising and public relations. Companies love the extra super-positive messaging, all for free.

- Affords a level of credibility that literally can't be bought. Brand advocates are more than just walking testimonials. They are living proof that you are the best.

- Provides pre-sold prospective customers. Advocate recommendations carry so much weight that they are worth much more than plain referrals. They deliver customers ready and committed to purchasing your product or service.

- Increases profits exponentially. Brand advocates are money-making machines for your business because they increase sales and decrease marketing costs.

For these reasons, brand advocacy is 12 out of 10!!

BRANDING YOURSELF: HOW TO DO SO IN FOUR EASY WAYS

If you're interested in branding your product or company, you may not be sure where to begin. The good news: I'm here to help. You can brand in many ways, but here I pare it down to four ways to help you start:

Branding by association

This way involves hanging out with and being seen with people who are very much higher than you in your particular niche.

Branding by achievement

This way repurposes your previous achievements.

Branding by testimonial

This way makes use of the testimonials that you receive but have likely never used.

Branding by WOW

A WOW is the pleasantly unexpected, the equivalent of going the extra mile. The easiest and most certain way to WOW people is to tell them that you've written a book. To discover how you can write a book of own, go to www.BrandingSmallBusinessForDummies.com.

Happiness: How to Experience the "Real Deals"

MARCI SHIMOFF

I was 41 years old, stretched out on a lounge chair by my pool and reflecting on my life. I had achieved all that I thought I needed to be happy.

You see, when I was a child, I thought there would be five main things that would ensure that I'd be happy: a successful career helping people, a loving husband, a comfortable home, a great body, and a wonderful circle of friends. After years of study, hard work, and a few "lucky breaks," I finally had them all. (Okay, so my body didn't quite look like Halle Berry's—but four out of five isn't bad!) You think I'd have been on the top of the world.

But surprisingly I wasn't. I felt an emptiness inside that the outer successes of life couldn't fill. I was also afraid that if I lost any of those things, I might be miserable. Sadly, I knew I wasn't alone in feeling this way.

While happiness is the one thing we all truly want, so few people really experience the deep and lasting fulfillment that fills our soul. Why aren't we finding it?

Because, in the words of the old country western song, we're looking for happiness in "all the wrong places."

Looking around, I saw that the happiest people I knew weren't the most successful and famous. Some were married, some were single. Some had lots of money, and some didn't have a dime. Some of them even had health challenges. From where I stood, there seemed to be no rhyme or reason to what made people happy. The obvious question became: *Could a person actually be happy for no reason?*

I had to find out.

So I threw myself into the study of happiness. I interviewed scores of scientists, as well as 100 unconditionally happy people. (I call them the Happy 100.) I delved into the research from the burgeoning field of positive psychology, the study of the positive traits that enable people to enjoy meaningful, fulfilling, and happy lives.

What I found changed my life. To share this knowledge with others, I wrote a book called *Happy for No Reason: 7 Steps to Being Happy from the Inside Out*.

One day, as I sat down to compile my findings, all the pieces of the puzzle fell into place. I had a simple, but profound "a-ha"—there's a continuum of happiness:

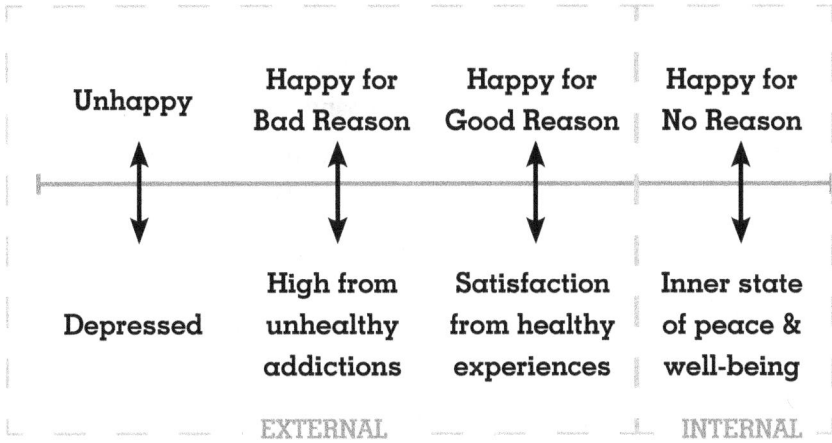

Unhappy: We all know what this means: life seems flat. Some of the signs are anxiety, fatigue, feeling blue or low—your "garden-variety" unhappiness. This isn't the same as clinical depression, which is characterized by deep despair and hopelessness that dramatically interferes with your ability to live a normal life, and for which professional help is absolutely necessary.

Happy for Bad Reason: When people are unhappy, they often try to make themselves feel better by indulging in addictions or behaviors that may feel good in the moment but are ultimately detrimental. They seek the highs that come from drugs, alcohol, excessive sex, "retail therapy," compulsive gambling, over-eating, and too much television-watching, to name a few. This kind of "happiness" is hardly happiness at all. It is only a temporary way to numb or escape our unhappiness through fleeting experiences of pleasure.

Happy for Good Reason: This is what people usually mean by happiness: having good relationships with our family and friends, success in our careers, financial security, a nice house or car, or using our talents and strengths well. It's the pleasure we derive from having the healthy things in our lives that we want.

Don't get me wrong. I'm all for this kind of happiness! It's just that it's only half the story. Being Happy for Good Reason depends on the external conditions of our lives—these conditions change or are lost, our happiness usually goes too. Relying solely on this type of happiness is where a lot of our fear is stemming from these days. We're afraid the things we think we need to be happy may be slipping from our grasp.

Deep inside, I think we all know that life isn't meant to be about getting by, numbing our pain, or having everything "under control." True happiness doesn't come from merely collecting an assortment of happy experiences. At our core, we know there's something more than this.

There is. It's the next level on the happiness continuum—Happy for No Reason.

Happy for No Reason: This is true happiness—a state of peace and well-being that isn't dependent on external circumstances.

Happy for No Reason isn't elation, euphoria, mood spikes, or peak experiences that don't last. It doesn't mean grinning like a fool 24/7 or experiencing a superficial high. Happy for No Reason isn't an emotion. In fact, when you are Happy for No Reason, you can have *any* emotion—including sadness, fear, anger or hurt—but you still experience that underlying state of peace and well-being.

When you're Happy for No Reason, you *bring* happiness to your outer experiences rather than trying to *extract* happiness from them. You don't need to manipulate the world around you to try to make yourself happy. You live from happiness, rather than *for* happiness.

This is a revolutionary concept. Most of us focus on being Happy for Good Reason, stringing together as many happy experiences as we can, like beads in a necklace, to create a happy life. We have to spend a lot of time and energy trying to find just the right beads so we can have a "happy necklace".

Being Happy for No Reason, in our necklace analogy, is like having a happy string. No matter what beads we put on our necklace—good, bad or indifferent—our inner experience, which is the string that runs through them all, is happy, and creates a happy life.

Happy for No Reason is a state that's been spoken of in virtually all spiritual and religious traditions throughout history. The concept is universal. In Buddhism, it is called causeless joy; in Christianity, the kingdom of Heaven within; and in Judaism it is called *ashrei*, an inner sense of holiness and health. In Islam it is called *falah*, happiness and well-being; and in Hinduism it is called *ananda*, or pure bliss. Some traditions refer to it as an enlightened or awakened state.

So how can you be Happy for No Reason?

Science is verifying the way. Researchers in the field of positive psychology have found that we each have a "happiness set-point," that determines our level of happiness. No matter what happens, whether it's something as exhilarating as winning the lottery or as challenging as a horrible accident, most people eventually return to their original happiness level. Like your weight set-point, which keeps the scale hovering around the same number, your happiness set-point will remain the same **unless you make a concerted effort to change it.** In the same way you'd crank up the thermostat to get comfortable on a chilly day, you actually have the power to reprogram your happiness set-point to a higher level of peace and well-being. The secret lies in practicing the habits of happiness.

Some books and programs will tell you that you can simply decide to be happy. They say just make up your mind to be happy—and you will be.

I don't agree.

You can't just decide to be happy, any more than you can decide to be fit or to be a great piano virtuoso and expect instant mastery. You can, however, decide to take the necessary steps, like exercising or taking piano lessons—and by practicing those skills, you can get in shape or give recitals. In the same way, you can become Happy for No Reason through practicing the habits of happy people.

All of your habitual thoughts and behaviors in the past have created specific neural pathways in the wiring in your brain, like grooves in a record. When we think or behave a certain way over and over, the neural pathway is strengthened and the groove becomes deeper—the way a well-traveled route through a field eventually becomes a clear-cut path. Unhappy people tend to have more negative neural pathways. This is why you can't just ignore the realities of your brain's wiring and *decide* to be happy! To raise your level of happiness, you have to create new grooves.

Scientists used to think that once a person reached adulthood, the brain was fairly well "set in stone" and there wasn't much you could do to change it. But new research is revealing exciting information about the brain's neuroplasticity: when you think, feel and act in different ways, the brain changes and actually rewires itself. You aren't doomed to the same negative neural pathways for your whole life. Leading brain researcher Dr. Richard Davidson, of the University of Wisconsin says, "Based on what we know of the plasticity of the brain, we can think of things like happiness and compassion as skills that are no different from learning to play a musical instrument or tennis .... it is possible to train our brains to be happy."

While a few of the Happy 100 I interviewed were born happy, most of them learned to be happy by practicing habits that supported their happiness. That means wherever you are on the happiness continuum, it's entirely in your power to raise your happiness level.

In the course of my research, I uncovered 21 core happiness habits that anyone can use to become happier and stay that way. You can find all 21 happiness habits at www.HappyForNoReason.com

Here are a few tips to get you started:

1. **Incline Your Mind Toward Joy.** Have you noticed that your mind tends to register the negative events in your life more than the positive? If you get ten compliments in a day and one criticism, what do you remember? For most people, it's the criticism. Scientists call this our "negativity bias" — our primitive survival wiring that causes us to pay more attention to the negative than the positive. To reverse this bias, get into the daily habit of consciously registering the positive around you: the sun on your skin, the taste of a favorite food, a smile or kind word from a co-worker or friend. Once you notice something positive, take a moment to savor it deeply and feel it; make it more than just a mental observation. Spend 20 seconds soaking up the happiness you feel.

2. **Let Love Lead.** One way to power up your heart's flow is by sending loving kindness to your friends and family, as well as strangers you pass on the street. Next time you're waiting for the elevator at work, stuck in a line at the store or caught up in traffic, send a silent wish to the people you see for their happiness, well-being, and health. Simply wishing others well switches on the "pump" in your own heart that generates love and creates a strong current of happiness.

3. **Lighten Your Load.** To make a habit of letting go of worries and negative thoughts, start by letting go on the physical level. Cultural anthropologist Angeles Arrien recommends giving or throwing away 27 items a day for nine days. This deceptively simple practice will help you break attachments that no longer serve you.

4. **Make Your Cells Happy.** Your brain contains a veritable pharmacopeia of natural happiness-enhancing neurochemicals — endorphins, serotonin, oxytocin, and dopamine — just waiting to be released to every organ and cell in your body. The way that you eat, move, rest, and even your facial expression can shift the balance of your body's feel-good-chemicals, or "Joy Juice", in your favor. To dispense some extra Joy Juice — smile. Scientists have discovered that smiling decreases stress hormones and boosts happiness chemicals, which increase the body's T-cells, reduce pain, and enhance relaxation. You may not feel like it, but smiling — even artificially to begin with — starts the ball rolling and will turn into a real smile in short order.

5. **Hang with the Happy.** We catch the emotions of those around us just like we catch their colds — it's called emotional contagion. So it's important to make wise choices about the company you keep. Create appropriate boundaries with emotional bullies and "happiness vampires" who suck the life out of you. Develop your happiness "dream team" — a mastermind or support group you meet with regularly to keep you steady on the path of raising your happiness.

"Happily ever after" isn't just for fairytales or for only the lucky few. Imagine experiencing inner peace and well-being as the backdrop for everything else in your life. When you're Happy for No Reason, it's not that your life always looks perfect — it's that, however it looks, you'll still be happy!

By Marci Shimoff. Based on the New York Times bestseller *Happy for No Reason: 7 Steps to Being Happy from the Inside Out*, which offers a revolutionary approach to experiencing deep and lasting happiness. The woman's face of the *Chicken Soup for the Soul* series and a featured teacher in *The Secret*, Marci is an authority on success, happiness, and the law of attraction. To order *Happy for No Reason* and receive free bonus gifts, go to www.happyfornoreason.com/mybook.

Sex, Love and Relationships

DR. JOHN GRAY

Just as great sex is important to lasting love, good health is important to sex and relationships. About 12 years ago, I cured myself of early stage Parkinson's disease. The doctors were amazed, but my wife was even more amazed. She noted that our relationship and sex life had become dramatically better. It turns out that the natural supplements I used to reverse Parkinson's can also make you more attentive and loving in your relationship. At that point, I realized that good relationship skills alone were not enough to sustain love and passion for a lifetime.

I shared many insights gained from my 40 years' experience as a marriage counselor and coach in *Men Are From Mars, Women Are From Venus*. And while my insights go a long way towards helping men and women understand and support each other, good communication skills alone are not always enough. For better relationships, we not only need to be healthy, but we must also experience optimum brain function.

If you are tired, depressed, anxious, not sleeping well, or in pain, then certainly romantic feelings will become a thing of the past. My recovery from Parkinson's revealed to me the profound connection between the quality of our health and our relationships. This insight has motivated me, over the past twelve years, to research the secrets of optimum health as a foundation for lasting love.

These are health secrets that are generally not explored in medical school. In medical school, doctors are indoctrinated into the culture of examining the symptoms, identifying the sickness, and prescribing a drug to treat that sickness. They learn very little about how to be healthy or to sustain successful relationships.

There are no university courses entitled "Better Nutrition For Better Sex". Drugs sometimes save lives, but they also have negative side effects that do little to preserve the passion in a relationship. Ideally, drugs should be used as a last resort and 90 % of our health plan should be drug free. From this perspective, the heath care crisis, as well as our high rate of divorce in America, is indirectly caused by our dependence on doctors and prescription drugs.

Most people have not even considered that taking prescribed drugs (even for the small stuff) can weaken their relationships, which in turn makes them more vulnerable to more disease. For example, if you are feeling depressed or anxious, a drug may numb your pain, but it does nothing to help you correct the cause of your problem. It can even prevent you from feeling your natural motivation to get the emotional support you need. In a variety of ways, our common health complaints are all expressions of two major conditions: our lack of education to identify and support unmet gender-specific emotional needs; and our lack of education to identify and support unmet gender-specific nutritional needs.

With an understanding of natural solutions that have been around for thousands of years, drugs are not needed to treat many common complaints. Some symptoms like low energy, weight gain, allergies, hormonal imbalance, mood swings, poor sleep, indigestion, lack of focus, ADD and ADHD, procrastination, low motivation, memory loss, decreased libido, PMS, vaginal dryness, muscle and joint pain, or the lack of passion in life and/or our relationships can be treated drug-free. By using drugs (even over-the-counter drugs) to treat these common complaints, our bodies and relationships are weakened, making us more vulnerable to bigger and more costly health challenges like cancer, diabetes, heart disease, auto-immune disease, dementia, and Alzheimer's. In simple terms, by handling the easy stuff (the common complaints) without doctors and drugs, we can protect ourselves from the big stuff (cancer, heart disease, dementia, etc.) We can be healthy and also enjoy lasting love and passion in our personal lives.

Even if you are taking anti-depressants or hormone replacement therapy, sometimes all it takes to stop treating the symptom is to directly handle the cause. With specific mineral orotates (something most people have never heard of) or omega three oil from the brains of salmon, your stress levels immediately drop and you begin to feel happy and in love again.

For every health challenge, we have explored the effects on our relationships, with as well as natural remedies that can sometimes produce immediate positive results. You can find these natural solutions to common health complaints for free at my website: www.MarsVenus.com.

What they don't teach in medical school is how to be healthy and happy without the use of drugs or hormone replacement. By refusing drugs and taking responsibility for your health, a wealth of new possibilities can become available to you. We are designed to be healthy and happy, and it is within our reach if we commit to increasing our knowledge.

New research regarding the brain differences in men and women reveals how specific nutritional supplements, combined with gender-specific relationship and self-nurturing skills, can stimulate the hormones of health, happiness and increased energy. Over the past 10 years in my healing center in California, I witnessed how natural solutions coupled with gender-specific relationship skills could solve our common health complaints without drugs. By addressing these common complaints without prescribed drugs, not only do we feel better, but our relationships have the potential to improve dramatically.

Ultimately the cause of all our common complaints is higher stress levels. Researchers around the world all agree that chronic stress levels in our bodies provide a basis for any and all disease to take hold. An easy and quick solution for lowering our stress reactions is specific nutritional support combined with gender-smart relationship skills. Extra nutritional support is needed because stress depletes the body very quickly of essential nutrients. When a car engine is running more quickly, it uses fuel more quickly. When we are stressed, we need both extra nutrients and extra emotional support. Understanding what we need to take and where to get it requires education. Every week day at www.MarsVenus.com I have a live daily show where I freely answer questions and provide this much-needed new gender-specific insight.

At www.MarsVenus.com, we are happy to share what we have learned for creating healthy bodies and positive relationships. You can find a host of natural solutions for common complaints and feel confident that you have the power to feel fully alive with an abundance of energy and positive feelings that will enrich all your relationships.

The Greatest Weapon Against Cancer Is Knowledge

Every Cancer Is Different. Learn About Your Risk And Ways to Reduce It

MELANIE R. PALOMARES, M.D., M.S.

Cancer afflicts millions of people and takes hundreds of thousands of lives each year. In 2012, the World Health Organization (WHO) reported 14 million new cancer diagnoses and 8.2 million deaths—and that number is projected to rise in the coming years.[1] Statistics suggest that about 39 percent of men and women will be diagnosed with this disease at some point during their lifetime.[2] The good news is that, today, early

1 World Health Organization Staff, "WHO | Cancer." World Health Organization, 2015. Web. http://www.who.int/mediacentre/factsheets/fs297/en/

2 National Cancer Institute Staff, "SEER Stat Fact Sheets: Cancer of Any Site." National Cancer Institute, 2013. Web. https://seer.cancer.gov/statfacts/html/all.html

detection and specialized treatment for different types of cancer can make all the difference.

Cancer used to be the disease that no one talked about—and, unfortunately, that meant that people at risk didn't even know about their family's medical history. Even today, there's a stigma surrounding cancer patients. In an article for *Cancer World*, the principal periodical of the European School of Oncology, Associate Editor Anna Wagstaff gives a harrowing report of the way societies around the world view cancer:

"Fears that the disease may be infectious can result in people being shunned by friends and neighbours (sic) and excluded from the community. Fears that it is hereditary can ruin the marriage chances of those with a mother or father known to have had cancer. Whole families can find themselves impacted, which can then put intolerable strains on relationships, leaving people with cancer even more isolated."[3]

The good news is that we are far more educated on the matter than we used to be. Today we have a wealth of information available via social media and the internet. The challenge is the quality of information available from such sources, which are not always subject to medical peer review. This has led to more awareness, and there have been more discoveries about lifestyle and environmental risk factors, which may be modified to improve cancer risk.

Studies have shown that the more accurate information one has, the better chance one has to maintain their health. In general, you are far more likely to survive a bout with cancer if you catch it at an early stage. For instance, Mayo Clinic reports the survival rate for colorectal cancer is 90% if it is caught early, although it is the second deadliest cancer in the United States, when all stages

---

3 World Health Organization Staff, "WHO | Cancer." World Health Organization, 2015. Web. http://www. Anna Wagstaff, "Stigma: Breaking the Vicious Cycle." Cancer World, 2013. Web. http://www.cancerworld.org/Articles/Issues/55/July-August-2013/Patient-Voice/602/Stigma-breaking-the-vicious-cycle.html

are considered.[4]

This information may motivate you to pursue cancer screenings, but you should know that those come with their own set of risks. For one thing, screening tests are not 100% reliable. Even when they are conducted by medical professionals you know and trust, the possibility of a false-positive or false-negative result exists. Beyond that, some testing procedures come with their own immediate hazards. Colonoscopies, for example, carry some risk of damaging the lining of the colon.[5] Therefore, it is important to pursue to proper type and frequency of screening for your level of cancer risk.

By far, the best defenses against cancer are prevention and proactivity. The National Cancer Institute estimates that as many as 50-75% of cancer fatalities in the United States are caused by negative lifestyle choices, like smoking, lack of exercise, or poor diet.[6] Just by living a healthy lifestyle, you can reduce your chances of contracting cancer dramatically.

That said, it is most important to know how prone you are to the disease. If the disease runs in your family, or if you think that you may have had an exposure that may increase your risk of developing cancer (examples of such risk factors are discussed throughout this chapter), you need not feel helpless. Your first step is to talk with an oncologist or a general physician with specific training and experience in understanding cancer risk factors to perform an accurate risk assessment. From there, you can obtain personalized cancer screening recommendations tailored to your level of risk. You can also learn about a variety of different precautions that you can take to minimize

---

4 Sharon Theimer, "Mayo Clinic Expert Shares Five Things to Know About Colorectal Cancer." Mayo Clinic News Network, 2016. Web. http://newsnetwork.mayoclinic.org/discussion/mayo-clinic-expert-shares-5-things-to-know-about-colorectal-cancer/

5 National Cancer Institute, "Cancer Screening Overview." National Cancer Institute, 2016. Web. https://www.cancer.gov/about-cancer/screening/patient-screening-overview-pdq

6 National Cancer Institute, NIH, DHHS. Cancer Trends Progress Report – 2011/2012 Update. Bethesda; 2012.

your chances of developing any form of cancer. It all comes down to having a keen knowledge of your personal history and knowing exactly what your body needs at any given time in your life, based on your age and occurrences in your life.

EVALUATING YOUR RISKS

When evaluating and minimizing your risk of developing cancer, it is important to note that one size does not fit all. Each form of cancer comes with a specific and distinct set of risk factors, variables that make you more or less susceptible to cancer development. In general, risk factors for cancer can be filed under two different classifications: genetic and environmental.

Genetic Risk Factors Are Inborn

Those with family histories of cancer, or those who inherit mutated genes from their parents, often have a relatively high chance of developing cancer. By nature, genetic risks are immutable and unalterable; we cannot, after all, change the way we were born. However, it is still important to recognize how your genes affect your chances of developing cancer, so that you may take appropriate preventive measures.

Environmental Risk Factors Are a Product of Nurture

These risk factors revolve around the characteristics of your living area, such as the climate (eg. sun exposure), the quality of the air you breathe, and the food you consume. Unlike genetic factors, environmental factors are, to some extent, subject to change. However, these changes may or may not be within your control, depending on what your living options are and whether you can afford to move.

In general, while there are many types and subtypes of cancer, all associated with different risk factors, screening, treatment, and prevention, in this chapter I will focus on the four most common cancers in the U.S.: breast and gynecologic cancers, colon cancer, lung cancer, and prostate cancer. These "Big Four" account for over 50% of all the cancers that occur in Americans.

BREAST AND GYNECOLOGIC CANCERS

From birth, sex hormones play an instrumental role in your body's growth, maturity and fertility. After you mature, your reproductive health is largely dependent on how well your body maintains the balance between estrogens and androgens. The enzyme aromatase plays a particularly vital part in a woman's reproductive health, breaking down larger hormones in the breasts and ovaries. This is important to note because breast cancer, like most gynecologic cancers, is hormone-driven.

The most important factors in determining breast cancer risk are gender and age. Since breast cancer growth is facilitated by the presence of female hormones, it serves to reason that the illness predominately affects women (but not only women). It also follows that breast cancer is most likely to develop post-maturity, when the body's hormonal activity reaches its peak. This is also the case for most ovarian and uterine cancers. On the other hand, cervical cancer is more likely to occur in young women, particularly those with more sexual activity, though the availability of human papilloma virus (HPV) vaccines will likely change the epidemiology of that disease as they become more commonly used for cancer prevention in girls and young women.

With breast and gynecologic cancers, despite popular belief, the role of inheritance is relatively minor. Although a family history of breast and/or ovarian cancer does make it more likely that you will develop one of these diseases, studies show that less than 15-20% of diagnosed breast cancer patients in America have immediate relatives with the same affliction,[7] and only about 5-10% have a strong family history of breast and/or ovarian cancer associated with a high cancer susceptibility genetic mutation. The most well-known examples are inherited mutations in the BRCA1 or BRCA2 genes, which are associated with the Hereditary Breast and Ovarian Cancer (HBOC) syndrome. Yet other cancer susceptibility genetic mutations, specifically mutations the DNA mismatch repair genes, are associated with a high risk of uterine and ovarian cancer with colon cancer, rather than breast cancer, in an entirely different inheritable entity called Lynch syndrome. In addition, there are gene mutations that carry only an intermediate elevation in risk for developing breast cancer, such as inherited mutations in a gene called PTEN, which are also associated with uterine cancer, thyroid cancer, and colon polyps as part of a less common familial entity called Cowden's syndrome. While there are even a few more familial syndromes that have been described to be associated with breast and/or gynecologic cancer, cervical cancer appears to be related to HPV infection as an environmental risk, with little to no relation to inheritance.

In addition to family history, you should also look into your personal history; breast cancer is more likely to happen in women who had their first period before age 12, as well as those who went through menopause relatively late.[8] The standard use of mammograms for breast cancer screening since the 1980s has shifted this disease to one that is more often caught early, except in younger women who may not have started regular screening yet. Two points

---

7 breastcancer.org Staff, "U.S. Breast Cancer Statistics." breastcancer.org, 2016. Web. http://www.breastcancer.org/symptoms/understand_bc/statistics

8 Mayo Clinic Staff, "Symptoms and Causes – Breast Cancer." Mayo Clinic, 2016. Web. http://www.mayoclinic.org/diseases-conditions/breast-cancer/symptoms-causes/dxc-20207918

follow from this trend: 1) women who have had findings of changes that occur prior to the development of a full cancer have an opportunity for medical prevention, and 2) it is particularly important to understand a woman's cancer risk in order to adjust screening recommendations to given high-risk women the same opportunity for early detection.

Lastly, diet and physical activity appear to play an important role in the development of these cancers. Obesity has been particularly associated with breast and uterine cancer. In addition, excessive alcohol use has been linked to breast cancer risk, particularly in premenopausal women.

COLORECTAL CANCERS

Colorectal cancers originate in the colon and rectum. The term "colorectal cancer" refers the most common of the cancers that develop within the human digestive tract. Colorectal cancers share a variety of causes and risk factors. One of them is chronic inflammation, as is seen in individuals with a history of the chronic inflammatory bowel diseases (IBD), Crohn's Disease or Ulcerative Colitis. Chronic inflammation can lead to the development of dysplasia, abnormally structured cells in the colon. Dysplastic cells often contain somatic, or non-inherited genetic mutations that are acquired after birth, which have the potential to develop into cancer cells over time.

Also, like breast and ovarian cancers, colorectal cancers have a familial component. In fact, there are some hereditary conditions that increase their carriers' propensity towards colorectal cancer. One such condition is Lynch syndrome, which was mentioned in the previous section, because of its association with uterine and ovarian cancers as well. Another syndrome is called familial adenomatous polyposis (FAP), an inherited condition that causes multiple polyps to grow in the patient's large intestine.[9] There are additional familial syndromes that have been described to be associated with colorectal cancers. These, as well as more detail about other cancer genetics syndromes, may be found at my website, www.caprevinc.org.

Diet is also thought to play a role in colon cancer, with certain elements, such as adequate folate and fiber intake, appearing to take an important role in minimizing risk.[10] Diets that include lots of vegetables, fruits, and whole grains have also been linked with a decreased risk of colon cancer. Dietary fat has been linked to a higher risk of colon cancer, as well as tobacco and alcohol use. The American Institute for Cancer Risk (AICR) estimates that 45% of colon cancers are preventable through diet, staying a healthy weight, and being physically active.[11]

LUNG CANCER

In general, lifestyle and environmental factors play the largest role in the development of lung cancer. This is an important point, in that lung cancer is the most common cause of cancer death in the United States, yet its risk factors are largely modifiable. Thus, it is important to understand these risks so that you can make the best choices for yourself and your family.

While tobacco use is the most well known risk factor, an additional major contributing factor is the exposure to secondhand smoke, or smoke expelled from used cigarettes and tobacco pipes. The American Cancer Society has

---

9 Al-Sukhni W, Aronson M, Gallinger S. "Hereditary colorectal cancer syndromes: familial adenomatous polyposis and lynch syndrome." Surg Clin North Am. 2008 Aug;88(4):819-44, vii. doi: 10.1016/j.suc.2008.04.012.

10 Giovannucci E, Willett WC. "Dietary factors and risk of colon cancer." Ann Med. 1994 Dec;26(6):443-52.

11 http://www.aicr.org/press/press-releases/preventing-colon-cancer-6-steps.html?referrer=https://www.google.com/

shown that secondhand smoke is even more toxic and carcinogenic than the vapor taken in by smokers themselves.[12] Because of this, the risk of lung cancer is relatively high for those who live or work around chronic smokers. Smoking and other tobacco use, such as chewing tobacco, also increases the risk for aerodigestive cancers, such as cancers of the oral cavity, throat, esophagus, and stomach. And because tobacco products can be excreted in the urine, tobacco use is also associated with kidney and bladder cancer.

Another large contributing factor to lung cancer is radon poisoning. Radon is a colorless, odorless substance that spawns from the natural decay of uranium in soil. Commonly, homes, particularly those in suburban or rural areas, can build up large quantities of radon over time as it rises up from the soil and seeps through cracks and flaws in the foundation. This is more common than you might think; in fact, it's responsible for roughly 21,000 lung cancer deaths each year, making it the second largest contributor to lung cancer behind tobacco.[13]

Asbestos is another major environmental factor associated with lung cancer. Asbestos poisoning is associated with a specific kind of lung cancer called mesothelioma. Since the 1980s, several laws have been passed in this country to restrict the availability and usage of asbestos in architecture. In spite of this, we still see a steady number of new mesothelioma diagnoses each year—about 3,000 annually, as estimated by the Mesothelioma Center.[14]

---

12 American Cancer Society, "Health Risks of Secondhand Smoke." ACS, 2015. Web. http://www.cancer.org/cancer/cancercauses/tobaccocancer/secondhand-smoke

13 Janet McCabe, "For peace of mind, add 'test for radon' to your 2016 to-do list." EPA Connect, 2016. Web.https://blog.epa.gov/blog/2016/01/test-for-radon/

14 The Mesothelioma Center, "Mesothelioma - Overview of Malignant Mesothelioma Cancer." asbestos.org, 2016. Web. https://www.asbestos.com/mesothelioma/

PROSTATE CANCER

Prostate cancer is the most common cancer occurring in American men, aside from skin cancer.[15] In 2016 alone, 26,120 American men were reported to have died from this affliction. In fact, one in seven men will be diagnosed with prostate cancer in their lifetime. Like breast and gynecologic cancers, prostate cancer is largely influenced by hormones; the difference, of course, is that it feeds off of androgens, male hormones, rather than estrogens.

Age is also a risk factor. Prostate cancer is seldom diagnosed in men younger than 40, and roughly 60% of cases are diagnosed in men at least 65 years of age.[16] Heredity and genes also play a role in prostate cancer development, although no highly penetrant cancer susceptibility genes have been described to date, unlike with breast, gynecologic, and colorectal cancers. Nevertheless, men who are closely related to prostate cancer patients are twice as likely to develop it themselves. The risk heightens even further if a man has more than one affected relative.

CANCER SCREENING

Cancer screening methods range from physical exam or self-exam to blood tests and specialized x-rays, such as mammograms, or procedures, such as colonoscopies. These methods are recommended to be performed at different frequencies depending upon age, family history, and other risk factors.

Concerns about false positive results, which can lead to unnecessary tests

---

15 Rebecca L. Siegel, Kimberly D. Miller and Ahmedin Jemal, "Cancer Statistics, 2016." CA: A Cancer Journal for Clinicians, 2016. Web. http://onlinelibrary.wiley.com/doi/10.3322/caac.21332/full

16 Prostate Cancer Foundation, "Prostate Cancer FAQs." Web. http://www.pcf.org/site/c.leJRIROrEpH/b.5800851/k.645A/Prostate_Cancer_FAQs.htm

and patient anxiety, as well as to overdiagnosis and overtreatment, has led to widespread controversy regarding different screening techniques. In addition, due to concerns about health care costs, cancer screening policies differ from country to country. This is why different guidelines are often offered by different medical organizations, which unfortunately leads to confusion for both consumers and health care professionals.

It is for this reason that I highly recommend seeking the advice of a physician with specific training and experience in understanding cancer risk factors to perform an accurate risk assessment. From there, you can obtain personalized recommendations specified to your risk level. Resources for determining your general category of cancer risk and, if appropriate, how to find a referral to a qualified health care professional near you can be found at my website, www.capревinc.org. Webinars on this topic are in development and will be available at that site as well.

REDUCING YOUR RISK

While cancer screening can help with early detection of cancer, which does improve outcomes with cancer treatment, as mentioned earlier in this chapter, it is important to remember that you have the power to help mitigate your chances of developing cancer in the first place (or getting it again, if you are a cancer survivor). Fighting the disease is a matter of recognizing what you can and cannot control, and focusing on what you can control. Your personal choices on a day-to-day basis can make a huge difference in your personal war against cancer, and you cannot go into battle without knowing what the consequences of those choices are.

LIFESTYLE INTERVENTIONS

A balanced, careful diet is key to fighting cancer. The influence of your food intake on your cancer risk cannot be overstated. Some foods actually have the potential to increase your risk of developing cancer, so it's vital to know what to eat, what to abstain from, and what to limit.

Diet: Plant-Based Foods

When it comes to prevention of and survivorship with cancer, fruits, vegetables and whole grains are the most desirable foods you can eat. Cancer.net educates patients about the link between excessive body fat and the development of several types of cancer, including the aforementioned colorectal cancer.[17] As such, your best bet is to eat foods that are low in fat and high in fiber. Plant-based food groups (vegetables, fruits, nuts, whole grains and legumes) all fit the bill. Fiber-rich foods in particular will help you along the way. Fiber is the broom of the digestive system, sweeping your intestines clean and keeping your digestive processes running at regular intervals. Because of this, fiber helps flush carcinogenic compounds out of your body, thus preventing cancer from growing.

Diet: Animal Products

While a plant-based diet is wholly important to cancer prevention, this does not mean you have to swear off meat and dairy altogether. You should, however, place significant limits on how much animal-based food you take in. Most people, especially Americans, consume far more meat than they should.

---

17 Cancer.net Editorial Board, "Obesity, Weight and Cancer Risk." Cancer.net, 2016. Web. http://www.cancer.net/navigating-cancer-care/prevention-and-healthy-living/obesity-and-cancer/obesity-weight-and-cancer-risk

In general, meat should not constitute more than a small fraction of the calories you take in per day. It's also important to recognize that some meats are better than others. Poultry and fish, for instance, are leaner and healthier alternatives to beef and pork. It's also a good idea to stay away from processed meats, like hot dogs and salami.

Physical Activity

Get moving! Exercise, particularly aerobic exercise, is an integral part of weight management, and by extension, cancer prevention. It is possible to reduce your risk for colorectal and breast cancer in particular with a regular exercise regimen. The AICR recommends sustained physical activity for at least 30 minutes a day.[18]

In addition to avoidance of obesity, which has been linked to an increasing number of different cancer types,[19] there are other benefits provided by regular exercise. For one thing, it keeps your metabolism running quickly and efficiently, which in turn will keep your weight at a healthy level. It also serves to strengthen your immune system, which plays an integral role in your body's defenses against cancer. Finally, regular exercise helps regulate your hormone levels which, as mentioned before, play a key role in the development of gynecologic cancers.

Stress Management

---

18 American Institute for Cancer Research, "Physical Activity Recommended for Preventing Cancer." AICR, 2016. Web. http://www.aicr.org/reduce-your-cancer-risk/recommendations-for-cancer-prevention/recommendations_02_activity.html

19 Béatrice Lauby-Secretan, Ph.D., Chiara Scoccianti, Ph.D., Dana Loomis, Ph.D., Yann Grosse, Ph.D., Franca Bianchini, Ph.D., and Kurt Straif, M.P.H., M.D., Ph.D., for the International Agency for Research on Cancer Handbook Working Group. Body Fatness and Cancer — Viewpoint of the IARC Working Group. N Engl J Med 2016; 375:794-798, August 25, 2016.

Chronic stress can affect body system functioning, particularly the immune system, and a weak immune system makes the body a more hospitable environment for cancer cells to grow. Stress also leads to release of a hormone called cortisol, which leads to truncal obesity, thereby leading to an increased risk of obesity-related cancers. Cortisol, along with other stress-related chemicals called catecholamines, has also been shown to directly facilitate cancer growth. Yet other stress hormones can inhibit a process called anoikis, which normally kills diseased cells and prevents them from spreading. Finally, chronic stress leads to increased production of growth factors that promote inflammation and new blood supply, which could potentially feed a developing cancer, as well as provide an environment for invasion and metastasis, or spread.[20]

While it is not realistic to avoid all sources of stress in our lives, it is possible to manage our relationship to external stressors. Mindfulness practices, such as meditation and yoga, can be very helpful in this regard. Getting adequate sleep not only supports successful stress management, but also allows to body to get the rest it needs to function well. Reading personal development books can help define knowledge and skills on how to manage situations that may be new or uncomfortable to us. Seeking the support of a mental health professional can be very helpful in identifying healthy ways to manage stress specific to your situation.

MEDICATIONS

If you are particularly worried about your susceptibility to cancer, there are a variety of cancer-suppressing medications that you can use. While some of them can be particularly potent cancer deterrents, they can be dangerous if

---

20 Myrthala Moreno-Smith, Susan K Lutgendorf, and Anil K Sood, Impact of stress on cancer metastasis. Future Oncol. 2010 Dec; 6(12): 1863–1881.

used improperly. As with any drug, consult your physician before taking any of these medications, and be sure that you know about all of the side effects and potential risks.

For those with family histories of colon cancer, the Food and Drug Administration (FDA) recommends Celecoxib, most often known under the brand name 'Celebrex.' It works by disrupting the formation of polyps in your digestive tract, thus preventing cancer cells from growing there. However, those with histories of heart problems should be wary of using Celebrex. It is classified as a Non-Steroidal Anti-Inflammatory Drug (NSAID), and some NSAIDs can heighten your risk of heart disease and stroke.[21] In some patients, it may also cause serious gastrointestinal problems, including stomach ulcers.[22] Some studies suggest that aspirin may be an alternative for colon cancer risk reduction.

For breast cancer, there is a class of drugs known as selective estrogen response modifiers, or SERMs for short. In general, they have two primary functions; firstly, they are designed to suppress the production of estrogen in certain body tissues, particularly those in the breast. Secondly, they take on the functions that estrogen would normally fulfill, thus enabling your body to function properly without facilitating breast cancer growth.

But, like NSAIDs, SERMs have their own set of risks. Tamoxifen, for instance, heightens your risk of developing blood clots and having a stroke (though this risk is still relatively small). Tamoxifen can also exacerbate the symptoms of menopause, including hot flashes and vaginal dryness.[23] Tamoxifen has been shown to slightly increase the risk of uterine cancer, but for women who have a high risk for developing breast cancer, this risk is

---

21 The Internet Drug Index, "Celebrex." RxList, 2011. Web. http://www.rxlist.com/celebrex-drug.htm

22 Omudhome Ogbru, "Celebrex Side Effects Center." RxList, 2016. Web. http://www.rxlist.com/celebrex-side-effects-drug-center.htm

23 National Cancer Institute, "Hormone Therapy for Breast Cancer." 2012. Web. http://www.cancer.gov/cancertopics/factsheet/Therapy/hormone-therapy-breast

outweighed by its breast cancer reduction effects.

For postmenopausal women, an aromatase inhibitor called exemestane (brand name: Aromasin) is another alternative for medical breast cancer risk reduction. This drug may also be associated with menopausal symptoms, and also is associated with bone loss and thus may not be a good option for women with osteoporosis or osteopenia.

Prostate cancer patients have their own class of hormonal suppressant preventive agents, called 5α-reductase inhibitors. Two medications fall into this class of drugs, finasteride (brand name: Proscar) and dutasteride (Avodart). Similar to SERMs, they work by suppressing the production of androgens in the patient's body, thus preventing a cancer from growing. But, just like SERMS, these drugs may come with side effects.

Despite their side effects, these medications can be very useful for individuals with a high risk for a specific cancer, which underscores the importance of talking with your doctor about cancer risk assessment. If you are found to be at high risk, a cancer prevention specialist may offer you consultation to see if the benefits of a particular drug far outweigh its side effects in your particular case.

SURGICAL INTERVENTION

Preventive surgery is a last resort, as it can be stressful, risky and exceedingly expensive. It should only be used if your risk of developing cancer is high enough to justify it.

The most common form of preventive surgery is a bilateral mastectomy, the removal of one or both of your breasts. A mastectomy is often used to remove cancerous tissue in the breast, but it can also be used proactively to prevent the growth of cancer in that area. While a mastectomy will reduce the risk of breast cancer by a huge margin, it will not eliminate the risk altogether. Also, as you would expect, there are a variety of unrelated risks that come with the mastectomy procedure. Like any surgery, a mastectomy can lead to scarring, disfigurement, infection in the surgical area and blood clots. As such, only patients with an exceedingly high susceptibility to breast cancer should consider this option.

Similarly, prophylactic bilateral salpingo-oophorectomy (removal of both fallopian tubes and ovaries to prevent ovarian cancer) or prophylactic colectomy (removal of all or part of the colon to prevent colon cancer) may be considered in special high-risk patients.

These are just a few of the methods you can use to snuff out cancer before it grows. In short, the best way to minimize your chance of developing cancer is to take care of yourself. Have a keen awareness of what your body needs on a day-to-day basis, and act accordingly. Watch what you eat, keep track of your physical activity, and consult an experienced physician. If you'd like to learn more about the various types of cancer and what you can do to lower your own risk, please visit www.caprevinc.org or call 844-PREV-INC.

In summary, reducing your risk of getting cancer is possible. Start by understanding your family medical history as well as lifestyle and environmental risk factors. Have a positive attitude, a strict sense of self-awareness, and the willingness to change what you can and accept what you can't but with a proactive plan to manage your risk.

If you would like to know more about Dr. Melanie R. Palomares, M.D., M.S., and Cancer Prevention, Inc. please visit http://www.caprevinc.org/.

One Step at a Time

Parents, Educators and Children with Autism Share their Success Stories

ANNE-CAROL SHARPLES

We all have aspirations and dreams for our children. Sometimes these expectations begin during our own childhoods as we dream about becoming parents. Sometimes the hopes and dreams do not begin until we look into the eyes of our newborn. No matter when the dream begins, no one dreams of autism. The diagnosis is a sucker-punch that leaves parents reeling and confused. Life quickly becomes complicated with all kinds of well-meant advice from professionals, family and strangers which include everything from medication to diet to the latest new therapy. This chapter does not offer advice on medicines, diet or therapies. The intention of this chapter is to uplift and inspire you. Perhaps you lay awake at night wondering, how I can fight the stigma related to the diagnosis. Maybe you cry, not because of who your child is, but because your child will not fit into the mold society expects. Please sit back and take a moment to learn about the successes of these autistic children and adults. It is with much love and respect that this chapter is dedicated to people on the autism spectrum as well as their families, teachers and caregivers.

SASHA

Sasha met all of her developmental milestones up until 22 months of age. It was then that the gregarious toddler fell silent. The daughter who was stringing two words together saying "What's this?" with inquisitive eyes vanished. Games and activities that Sasha once enjoyed no longer interested her. Eye contact became fleeting and she rarely responded to her name anymore. Sensing red flags, Sasha's parents Marjorie and Ryan began piecing the puzzle together. Shortly after, Sasha was diagnosed with autism. Devastated, but determined to bring back the vivacious child they once knew, the family began a courageous journey that would challenge every aspect of their personal relationships.

Investigating therapies, spending what seemed like hours on the phone and placing Sasha on waitlists left them disconcerted and worn out. Turning to one another for support, they drew upon each other's strengths and continued to map out the next steps in the journey. Together they discussed therapy options, and often reached for the other's hand when either one awoke panic stricken in the middle of the night, worried if they were doing the right thing.

Engaging Sasha in experiences and pulling her out of her shell that she so often retreated into became their undertaking. Sasha began Intensive Behavioral Intervention Therapy (IBI) on a daily basis. Family outings and activities took place every weekend. Rather than shielding Sasha from the world that overwhelmed her, her family wanted her to experience it in positive ways.

Sasha continued IBI until she turned four. It was then that Marjorie and Ryan registered her at the neighborhood school. Beginning kindergarten proved to be very challenging for Sasha and her family. The one-to-one therapy she'd been receiving each weekday was a stark contrast to the room filled with twenty-five boisterous children. IBI Therapy was usually quiet and controlled; the kindergarten classroom was anything but quiet! Sasha was overwhelmed and the first few weeks of school were traumatic for her. As Sasha entered the classroom each day a change would come over her. Her muscles tensed, arms and legs flailed, hands became fists and her jaw clamped shut. Sasha was in protective, fight mode. She was uncommunicative, confused and often distressed, making it impossible to participate in classroom activities. When the other children would sit in circle time and share their stories, she'd become increasingly agitated. Sasha's parents were quite concerned as she collapsed with exhaustion at the dinner table each evening, but they knew her adjustment would take time and vowed to continue taking her to school. What they did not know then, was that school would be the turning point for their daughter.

Marjorie and Ryan decided to use their beloved family outings as a way for Sasha to engage at school. They began to send in pictures of her with short anecdotes written on them. There were pictures of Sasha with her pet bird, at the pumpkin patch, visiting the zoo and opening presents on her birthday. On each of these pictures, Marjorie wrote about each day and what was occurring in the photograph. Over time, Sasha began to respond to these photos when her teacher shared them with her classmates during circle time. Slowly, with support from her teacher, Sasha began to sit for circle time. She'd become very excited when she saw a picture of herself. Sasha's teacher, Mrs. Watson, knew she wanted to share the stories of the pictures herself, so she would have Sasha stand beside her and share her stories through pointing and babbling. Sasha was beginning to communicate at school.

Mrs. Watson played a vital role in Sasha's success at school; for instance, she recognized that Sasha was overwhelmed by the large number of students in the class, so she assigned her a spot right next to her during circle time. She also introduced a visual schedule so that Sasha would know what to expect throughout her day. When there was an unanticipated disruption in her schedule, Mrs. Watson used an "Oops" card to demonstrate the change. Sasha began to communicate with Mrs. Watson by babbling and pointing to the pictures on her schedule. When she was hungry, she pointed to a picture of "snack." She even began to switch her schedule around to her preferred activities and would giggle while proudly showing Mrs. Watson the changes she had made. Sasha grew to love Mrs. Watson; she had a gentle tone of voice and made everyone feel welcome in her classroom. She made school fun for all of her students and her love for teaching shone through her interactions with the students. In addition to utilizing the photographs Sasha's parents sent in, she also recognized Sasha's love for books. Mrs. Watson provided her with a copy of the story she was reading to the class each day. Sasha could hold her book and look at the pictures while Mrs. Watson read aloud to the class. This was a simple yet effective way of keeping her engaged during story time.

Sasha was fortunate to have Mrs. Watson as her Senior Kindergarten teacher the following year. This is the year she began to speak. It began with a word mixed in with gibberish and pointing. It was easy enough to understand, so whoever Sasha was communicating with could model the appropriate language. Soon she began stringing two words together, then two became four so that "blah, blah backpack" became, "I want my backpack."

Sasha is now in first grade and loves school; she reads, writes and talks constantly. The other students adore Sasha because she is persistent, passionate and a joy to be around. She loves to share stories of family outings with her teachers and classmates, with or without photographs.

HENRY

When our son, Henry, was three years old, we were told that he'd never speak or be able to perform simple tasks. We watched, on pins and needles, as the developmental evaluator modeled the activity of stacking three blocks on top of each other and held our breath as she handed the blocks to Henry for him to duplicate what she'd done. Our hearts broke when he was unable to even attempt to stack them. After this evaluation, his father and I were told that Henry would need to be institutionalized. After the shedding of countless tears and multiple late night discussions, we knew that we would not put our son in an institution. We refused to give up hope that we could find a way to help Henry. We enrolled Henry in a school that offered special needs classrooms.

We were fortunate to find a wonderful group of teachers who worked tirelessly to see that Henry was able to function to the best of his ability. After two years in school, with the inclusion of daily therapy, he was able to communicate, albeit in a limited way. Henry never entered a mainstream classroom, but he has achieved multiple successes. The educators and assistants in Henry's special needs classrooms refused to accept the idea of can't. They repudiated the limitations that had been placed on Henry by various doctors and educational evaluators. They only saw what Henry could do and the sky was the limit as far as they were concerned.

Over the years Henry learned how to not only stack blocks, but to tie his shoes and dress himself. He will never hold a job or live by himself, but Henry has made huge strides from what we were originally told he would be able to accomplish. We know that institutionalization would not have been the best choice for Henry as he never would have progressed to the level that he is at today.

ABIGAIL

Here it was again, the dreaded block test. Abigail's grandmother, Eleanor, rolled her eyes as she watched the evaluator hand the blocks to Abigail. She knew Abigail would not stack the blocks or build the bridge the evaluator had shown her. Why are these blocks so important anyway she wondered? Abigail was four years old and had missed most of the developmental milestones. She was not yet speaking coherently; in fact, Abigail had little interest in speaking and seemed unconcerned if her needs were not met. She was absorbed by her own world and took little notice of anything occurring around her. Eleanor wondered if this was because Abigail's mother had abandoned her when she was eighteen months old. She suspected the troubles were compounded by issues in addition to abandonment and was not surprised by the diagnosis of autism. She was surprised when the healthcare professionals told her that Abigail would likely never speak or communicate because she was locked inside her own world. Institutionalization was mentioned, but quickly dismissed by Eleanor. She knew there was more for Abigail and held on to hope that she would find help for Abigail.

As it turned out, help was found during Abigail's first year of school. She started out at age five, a year behind most of the other children in the Junior Kindergarten class. Abigail's teachers and support staff read through the medical and behavioral evaluations and chose a course of action: Abigail was taught just as the other children were taught, with patience, love and repetition. Her teachers did not become frustrated when Abigail stared blankly and did not repeat the sounds they were asking her to make. Instead, they simply tried again the next day. Gradually, Abigail began to come out of her shell, appearing more aware and less self-absorbed. She haltingly began to repeat sounds, then words.

After two years of kindergarten, Abigail was speaking and able to communicate her needs and desires. Her comprehension moved more slowly; it was not until grade three that Abigail began to understand that she should take off her jacket when she felt warm. Her schoolwork moved slowly, as well. Her teachers spent extra time working with her each day and she worked with her grandmother and tutors in the afternoons and throughout summers.

Over the years, Abigail spent countless hours working after school with her tutors and teachers. Her grandmother worked tirelessly to see that Abigail reached her goals. Abigail graduated from high school and is now living on her own in an apartment with two other girls. She even has her dream job working at an amusement park she loved going to as a child.

MARIAH

My name is Mariah and I am twenty-one years old and I have autism. What autism means for me is that I am an excellent painter. I paint better than your average person does. I used to go to school, but now I am finished with school and can paint any time I want. This is very exciting for me because I love to paint; it's my favorite thing to do! My dad takes me and my paintings to art shows where we sell the paintings. My dad always says to do what you love and you will be happy.

MARIAH'S DAD

Mariah struggled with school. She is an excellent reader, but struggles with short-term memory and cannot recall recently taught basic math functions. She was teased often and never understood why the other kids didn't behave as she thought they should. She would often tell the other children what to do, an action that did not win her many friends. She didn't understand the rules of the playground and would push other kids off the swings when she wanted a turn. Her mother and I worried that she'd never be able to hold a job due to her lack of social skills and memory struggles. We wanted more for Mariah. We can provide for her financially, but wanted her life to have quality. We wanted Mariah to be joyful and content.

When she was in her first year of high school, Mariah took an art class and fell in love with painting. She loves the vivid colors and the feel of the paint. Her art teacher recognized that, not only did Mariah have a talent for painting, but that painting was restorative for Mariah. If Mariah was having a rough day at school, her teacher would bring her to the art room where she could calm herself with paint. Her mother and I were stunned at the artwork she brought home. Painting gives Mariah joy. She loves to go to art shows and speak with people about her paintings; she could talk about her paintings for hours! She has felt true success by giving enjoyment to others with her artwork. Since she is able to experience other people's reactions to her paintings, she is inspired to continue working on her craft. Mariah's struggles with interacting with other people evaporate when she speaks of her art. People may not understand Mariah's way of thinking, but they understand her art.

Art is the desire of a man to express himself, to record the reactions of his personality to the world he lives in. Amy Lowell, poet

LILY AND CHARLENE

Charlene will never forget the first day she met Lily. At that time, Lily's only way of communicating was to scream. Lily was four years old, an only child who lived in a low-income apartment with her father. At the time Charlene met her, Lily had received no prior intervention; she was a cautious girl who clung to her father's leg on that day in her apartment. While Lily's father was giving Charlene a snapshot of what the first four years of Lily's life had been like, Lily let it be known that she was displeased with the disruption to her routine. She screamed, climbed the furniture, and removed her clothing in protest. The volume of her screams pierced the air and her father worried that the neighbors would complain, yet again, about the noise. Her father explained that he had been unable to accomplish basics, such as getting Lily to sit in a chair to eat.

The years of struggle, both financial and emotional, wore on his face; he was desperate for help. His spirit was broken, beaten down by the everyday demands of life and compounded by his daughter's needs and his inability to understand her. Charlene desperately wanted to help and felt as though she were carrying a load of bricks as she walked away from their apartment, weighted down by the father's anguish for his daughter.

Charlene went to the school where she was employed as a support worker to speak with the principal about helping Lily. Principal Anderson's son is on the autism spectrum, so he related to the anguish Lily's father was experiencing. Plans were made and Lily began Junior Kindergarten the following week. To say that Lily's first day was exhausting for not only Lily, but also her dad and the staff would be an understatement. The five minute walk from their apartment building to the school took more than half an hour as Lily battled her father every step of the way. Upon arrival at school, it took another fifteen or so minutes for Lily's dad to convince her to enter the building. She made it to the threshold of the classroom and remained there all day long, screaming whenever anyone entered her space or tried to engage her. This continued for several weeks, and throughout that time Charlene persevered by remaining calm and respecting Lily's need for space. By doing this, Charlene gained Lily's trust along with the admiration of the classroom teacher and the staff within the school.

Charlene had a unique way of interacting with Lily; she understood that Lily's behavior was her only way of communicating. She treated Lily with dignity and respect and accepted her where she was. Charlene recognized how difficult school was for Lily and took baby-steps with her, acting as a guide who would remain with Lily until she was ready to go it alone. Over the weeks Lily moved from the threshold of the classroom door to learning how to sit inside the classroom, with Charlene at her side. This was accomplished with patience and kindness, but also with a song. "Row, Row, Row Your Boat" was sung to alert Lily that it was time to enter the classroom and sit down. Lily liked the song and began to request it by holding her hands out and rocking back and forth. Charlene found an old wooden boat and brought it into the classroom so that Lily could sit in the boat and rock it from side to side. This was a motivating experience for Lily since she loved to rock. It is from sitting in the boat that Lily learned how to sit in a chair.

Charlene shared the idea of singing the song with Lily's father. He began singing the song at home to alert Lily that it was time to sit down to eat. Her father was overjoyed when Lily joined him at the table, sat in a chair and shared a meal with him. Charlene was able to accomplish so much with Lily by taking the time to get to know and understand her. It is individuals like Charlene, who have an innate ability to be present and want to help, that make peoples' hearts smile. Lily's father's heart was smiling by the end of her Junior Kindergarten year as he found hope for his daughter's future.

CAITLIN

Mondays are the best. At least Caitlin thinks so because Monday is horseback riding day. Caitlin is fifteen years old and has been diagnosed with autism, in addition to several other health concerns. Caitlin does not have much energy and, as a general rule, does not enjoy exercise. However, she loves all things horse-related; she enthusiastically shows up for her horseback riding lesson and will brush her horse and clean out his stall with gusto. Not every day goes so well. Caitlin struggles when things do not go as she expects and some days Caitlin becomes irritated with her horse and kicks or even punches him out of frustration. Caitlin is working on developing patience, accommodating changes to routine and communicating with her horse without kicking or punching.

Her mother is thrilled with the life lessons, as well as the Hippotherapy Caitlin has received and has shared Caitlin's successes with her special needs classroom teacher, Mrs. McFray. Being quite perceptive, Mrs. McFray decided to explore Caitlin's interest in other animals. She learned that Caitlin has a passion for all animals; therefore, Mrs. McFray incorporated a classroom unit on animals and even obtained a grant to purchase several animals for her classroom. The animals, which include a turtle, a bunny, two guinea pigs and a hedgehog have been a huge hit with all of the students in the special needs classroom.

Caitlin's favorite is the bunny, Mr. Cuddles. She loves to feed him mint and watch him motor his way through the stalk. The students have learned that they cannot hold or pet an animal when they are angry because the animal will become frightened. Prickles, the hedgehog, rolls into a tight ball when she is scared or hears loud noises. Mrs. McFray believes that her students know exactly how Prickles feels. The students can only hold Prickles when they are quiet and calm; they are learning to self-regulate in order to interact with a classroom animal. The classroom pets are treasured by all; therefore the students are highly motivated to regulate their emotions. Because Mrs. McFray took the time to listen to Caitlin's mom, ponder what she heard, and explore options for incorporating animals in her classroom, all of the students have benefited. Mrs. McFray has a deep affection for her students and wants to offer each of them the best learning environment possible.

MILES

Hi, my name is Miles and I'm fourteen years old. I always knew there was something different about me, and it was confirmed when I was seven and told that I have Asperger's Syndrome. Fitting in at school, or anywhere else, has always been difficult for me. I wanted friends, but couldn't figure out how to make them. Things would start out okay, but after a while I noticed that my friends would not be around our usual hangouts. Even worse, when they'd see me they would turn their backs or walk away. I never understood what I'd done wrong. Having friends, then immediately losing them was the hardest part of school for me. The schoolwork was easy-peasy and I probably could've done it with my eyes closed. Recess was a nightmare. At least it was a nightmare until I met Mrs. Wiley and began attending the Program to Assist Social Thinking, aka PAST. I dedicate this story to her. It is due to Mrs. Wiley that I am where I am today.

I began attending PAST one day a week when I was in third grade and I liked it from the start. The best part of PAST is that it is a safe place where we can be ourselves and not worry about anything. You see, all of the kids who attend PAST have autism. And, all of the teachers are super cool and completely understand us. I feel comfortable in my own skin and I can be me when I'm there. Now, that doesn't mean that everything is fun and easy. My teachers challenge me all the time. They know exactly how far to push me and understand when I become frustrated. In fact, they taught me how to control my emotions. Mrs. Wiley, my parents, and my third grade teacher, Mrs. Smyth, would come up with goals I needed to work on at school and at home. So, one of the items my mom really wanted me to learn was how to ask her how her day was and to be genuinely interested in her response. One of the items my teacher wanted me to do was to greet her every morning. Each day I was rated on my performance and scores were tallied up weekly. Once I mastered these goals, other goals were set.

What makes PAST so much fun is that we do super-cool activities, like going rock climbing or to the aquarium that has sea life from around the world. Also, we have a Bearded Dragon in our class! In fact, Eragon, our Bearded Dragon, is such a popular guy, I don't think he is ever in his cage. He has a calming effect on all of us when we are upset. Another activity we do is sit on extremely cool bean bag chairs and do role plays. We also play games to learn about all sorts of barriers that prevent us from being social thinkers. One of my barriers is that I get stuck on what I want to do all of the time. At PAST we have to learn to work as a team and not just do what we want to do. We have a marble jar and each of us puts a marble in the jar when we are being social thinkers. Once the jar is full, we go on an outing; it could be eating at a neighborhood restaurant or checking out the largest indoor reptile zoo. We vote on it and decide. My teacher says we are working, but it feels more like fun than work!

I now realize that my friends used to avoid me as a result of me always wanting things my way. I wanted to be the boss of the whole shebang, from a game of soccer to only talking about what I wanted to talk about. Now I understand that it is important to let other people talk and to listen to them, even if I'm not all that interested. Mrs. Wiley and PAST have taught me how to interact with others and how to have a conversation. Now I know how to start and continue a conversation. PAST has taught me about the perspective of others. I used to think that everyone thought the same way I do. Well, I sure was surprised to find out this isn't so!

Anne Wiley retired from her role as a PAST Teacher in 2014 but continues to volunteer and contribute to the Autism Department at the TCDSB.

The Vegan Lifestyle Solution

Make the Connection Between Your Diet and Your Purpose

DAGMAR SCHOENROCK

When I was asked to write a chapter for The Authorities book series, my first thought was, "Me, an authority? I'm a compassionate vegan, not a scientist, not a nutritionist, nor do I have a Ph.D." Nonetheless, I realized that there is no authority outside oneself. I am my own authority on the life experiences that I've had, ones that took me from bison farmer to vegan. This transition was clearly a life lesson, showing me that I need to trust myself — to be my own authority. With this in mind, I am grateful to have the opportunity to share with you some of the facts that helped me return to my true vegan state of being.

Every day, in fact, I'm filled with love and gratitude for the many privileges I've been blessed with. My gratitude list is long and it begins with my parents. Thanks to them, I was raised in a country with many civil liberties, a solid economic base and a peaceful society. This wasn't by accident. I was graced with this life because my parents left their homeland and immigrated to the Canadian prairies for the sake of their children. They wanted us to grow up in a free society and live in peace, safe from the political unrest in Europe. From an early age, I knew and appreciated the value of protecting others, sacrificing for others, and peace.

This awareness played a role in how I lived my life even as a child. I would bring home stray cats and dogs, baby birds that had fallen out of their nests, or turtles trying to cross the road, asking my parents to help me reunite them with their mothers. In school, I brought home bullied classmates until the students intimidating them passed by, and they could safely walk home to their own mothers. In college, I participated in fundraising efforts for various charities to eradicate illnesses or poverty. Later, I became a Big Sister and continued with fundraising for various organizations. When I became a parent, I continued my peaceful efforts by donating to environmental and human rights groups, supporting our local green candidate in the elections, and becoming a Girl Guides leader.

I don't believe this involvement in my community makes me unique; I believe this is what connects me to all of you. Like most people, I have a goal to contribute, in some small way and through some small action, to a free and peaceful society where we can all live in harmony and peace. Regardless of our level of contribution to this cause, we are all connected with the common thread of wanting to make the world a better place. Just think of all of the people you personally know who want to make the world a better place — your parents, your family doctor, the leader of your spiritual and/or religious group, your local humane society, the volunteers in your local community, etc. And now think of all of the organizations around the world whose sole purpose it is to make the world a better place by standing up for social justice, animal rights, human rights, or environmental protection. It's quite exciting, isn't it? All of these people, working and volunteering to make the world a better place, often at a personal sacrifice.

So my question to you is this: If so many individuals and organizations are dedicating their free time, careers, or even lives to making the world a better place, why do we still not live in peace and freedom? It doesn't make sense, does it? Shouldn't this common thread of wanting to make the world a peaceful place lead to common solutions for our global issues? And if the solutions were identified, would you be willing to make the sacrifices necessary to make them happen?

That last question is the hardest one. A good analogy can be taken from the movie The Matrix. In the film, the lead character Neo is given a choice of two pills. The blue pill allows him to go to sleep and wake up the next morning believing whatever he likes. The red pill allows him to see the truth. As Neo's mentor Morpheus says, "You have to see it for yourself. After this, there is no turning back. Remember, all I'm offering is the truth, nothing more."

Would you be willing to take a risk and swallow the red pill that shows you the truth? What if you learned that affecting positive change for global issues relating to social justice, animal rights, human rights, and the environment could be as simple as food choices? By adopting a plant-based, vegan diet, we can have a profound effect in all of these areas. Vegan benefits are felt most immediately in our state of health but extend well beyond into improving the global issues that affect us all. As Will Tuttle, Ph. D., and author of The World Peace Diet states, "Mindful eating is the essential foundation of happiness and peace."

WHAT IS VEGANISM?

To understand the potential global impact of veganism, we should start with the definition of that term. Although the practice of veganism has been noted throughout history, the founder of the Vegan Society, Donald Watson, defined the term "vegan" in 1944 as we understand and use it today. In coining the word, he distinguished vegan beliefs and habits from those of vegetarians. Generally, vegetarians abstain from eating meat, whereas vegans reject meat and animal products in all forms. Not only do they not consume meat, dairy, eggs, or honey, true vegans do not use any clothing, accessories or objects made from an animal.

BODY, MIND, AND SPIRIT

The Body: Improved Physical Health

Before I delve into the far-reaching benefits of a vegan lifestyle, I will begin with the personal advantages it brings to individuals. It's easy to say a new lifestyle improves our body, mind and spirit, but our very nature compels us to seek proof, and rightly so. For years, both the medical and scientific communities have been working to provide data that backs up this claim.

Neal D. Barnard, M.D., renowned physician and president of the Physicians Committee for Responsible Medicine, provides some of the most recent data supporting this claim. Results from his clinical study showed health improved on all fronts for participants with a plant-based diet. According to his research, "People not only slim down, but also see their cholesterol levels plummet and their blood pressure fall. If they have diabetes, it typically improves and sometimes even disappears. Arthritis pains and migraines often vanish, and energy comes racing back. Sluggishness vanishes, and they look and feel radiant."

Those are amazing results, aren't they? The physical benefits of a vegan diet go even further than those addressed by Dr. Barnard. Studies also demonstrate a direct correlation between a meatless diet and a lower body mass index (BMI), which is a typical indicator of healthy weight and lack of fat on the body. The International Journal of Obesity reported a six-year study by scientists at the University of Oxford with 38,000 participants of varied eaters (vegetarians, vegans, meat-eaters and fish-eaters) and found vegans to have the lowest BMI by a significant margin.

This lower BMI translates into healthy weight loss. Eating vegan eliminates most of the unhealthy foods that tend to cause weight issues. Once you adopt a vegan lifestyle, you develop an affinity for new foods, and as your palate changes, so do your cravings. By making a wise choice for your body, you begin to feel more positive.

Another benefit that vegans find as a result of their lifestyle is improved energy levels. More and more professional athletes attest to this, and what better source is there than the people whose very careers depend on their energy and stamina? To name just a few, former Celtics player Robert Parish, famed World Series Champion Hank Aaron and gold medal Olympian Carl Lewis are all major advocates of the vegan lifestyle. Lewis says, "I've found that a person does not need protein from meat to be a successful athlete. In fact, my best year of track competition was the first year I ate a vegan diet. Moreover, by continuing to eat a vegan diet, my weight is under control, I like the way I look. (I know that sounds vain, but all of us want to like the way we look.) I enjoy eating more, and I feel great."

German strongman Patrik Baboumian is another successful career athlete following a vegan diet. At Toronto's 2013 Vegetarian Food Festival, he clearly disproved any belief that to be a strong athletic competitor you must consume quantities of meat when he carried a yoke weighing more than 1200 pounds across the stage.

Outside of maintaining a healthy weight, being vegan improves the body physically in other ways. Healthy skin is dependent on antioxidants like beta-carotene and vitamins A, C and E, which are found predominantly in fruits and vegetables. It follows naturally that vegans will receive an infusion of these as compared to non-vegans. The elimination of dairy plays a role as well. Many dairy-producing cattle are injected with the growth hormone IGF-1, which causes swelling, redness, and clogged pores in humans. Even ailments such as PMS, migraines, and allergies decrease significantly with a vegan lifestyle.

The Mind: Improved Mental Health

In a 2012 issue of Nutrition Journal, Bonnie Beezhold and Carol Johnson reported findings that being vegan definitively improves a person's mood. In their study, participants were divided into three groups: omnivores, fish-eaters and vegetarians. After two weeks, participants completed a "Profile of Mood States" questionnaire and a "Depression Anxiety and Stress Scale" questionnaire. What were the results? The vegetarian group showed significant improvements in their mood scores at the end of the two-week trial. The findings were of no surprise to researchers, who have long known that meat and poultry diets are high in arachidonic acid (omega 6), which is linked to clinical symptoms of depression.

It's important to note, however, that omega 6 is an essential fatty acid, meaning our body does not manufacture it but requires it for good health. To find a balanced omega intake, vegans turn to plant sources instead, such as walnuts, pecans, avocado, flaxseed oil and other plant oils. Not only do these omega sources recover any deficiency that not eating meat may cause, they are also the same sources of vitamins known to improve mood. In other words, you're not only removing dietary items known to cause depression, you're adding foods that have the benefit of improving mood – a double bonus!

The Spirit: Improved Emotional Health

The emotional benefits of a vegan lifestyle are closely tied to the physical benefits. The bottom line is this: if you don't feel well physically, you won't be happy. Constant aches and pains quickly turn good emotional health into general unhappiness. Who among us hasn't had this experience? A lifestyle with good health and nutrition at its core can't help but improve your mood. When you eat well, you feel well.

Veganism also provides an opportunity for us to achieve success. Making the transition is not without challenges, and doing so successfully leads to a sense of pride and self-satisfaction. Our emotional health is better when we have embraced something wholeheartedly, as you do when you properly adhere to a vegan lifestyle. Simply put, it feels good to improve yourself and to do good for animals too.

A new lifestyle means new friends as well: another boost for our emotional health. Having a passion for a cause helps us become more outgoing as we seek to share our knowledge and excitement. A good deed shared by many feels even better than a good deed managed alone.

BEYOND OURSELVES

Now that you know about the personal benefits of veganism, it's time to discuss what to many vegans is even more important: how a vegan lifestyle lets us look beyond ourselves to improve the world. Sound dramatic? It is! Just imagine that a change in your lifestyle can implement change for everyone!

The Environment

"The sixteen hundred dairies in California's Central Valley alone produce more waste than a city of 21 million people — that's more than the populations of London, New York and Chicago combined." — Gene Baur, co-founder and president of Farm Sanctuary.

In a report published by the Food and Agriculture Organization of the United Nations (FAO), we learn that meat production has quadrupled in the past 50 years. Today, farmed animals (animals raised for consumption such as cattle, pigs, chickens, ducks, turkeys, egg-laying hens and dairy cows) outnumber people by more than three to one. Initially, "21 million people," "quadrupled in the past 50 years" and "more than three to one" seem like insurmountable figures, don't they? They certainly don't come across as something to be dealt with in the day-to-day life of average people like us. The truth is, these figures are of great importance to each and every one of us, as they warn us of increased global warming, pollution, water scarcity, deforestation, land degradation, species extinction and world hunger.

Consider, for instance, the relationship between farmed animals and global warming. As most of us know, scientists have been studying the results and effects of global warming's rising temperatures, rising sea levels, melting icecaps and glaciers and shifting ocean currents and weather patterns for years. It's no surprise that they've determined global warming is one of the most serious environmental challenges we're facing. So how is the amount of farmed animals related to global warming? The fact is, farmed animals are responsible for 18 percent of the greenhouse gas emissions that contribute to global warming. Just think about that for a minute. If everyone were to adopt a vegan lifestyle, we would cut emissions by almost a fifth.

Another factor in the correlation between the high farmed-animal count and negative impacts on the environment is the amount of water used to maintain them. The organization People for the Ethical Treatment of Animals (PETA) reports that it takes more than 2,400 gallons of water to produce one pound of meat, while growing one pound of wheat only requires 25 gallons. Not only is animal farming a great drain on natural water supplies, it's a major source of water pollution as a result of the animal waste, antibiotics and hormones, chemicals from tanneries, fertilizers and pesticides and sediments from eroded pastures that are found in water run-off.

Expansion of farmed animal production is also a key element in deforestation. In Latin America, 70 percent of what was once forested land in the region is now used for pastures and feedcrops. Land once valued for creating oxygen, filtering pollutants and stabilizing the global climate has been turned over to the farmed-animal industry. The natural benefits of these forests are lost, and species native to them are rapidly becoming endangered or extinct. Stripping the planet's green spaces is literally affecting the chances of your survival.

Equally concerning is the potential for farmed animal populations to cause world hunger to worsen. As more and more societies become dependent on farmed animals for a significant portion of their diet, the demand for meat is growing too rapidly to keep up with. According to the World Watch Institute, if everyone received 25 percent of their needed daily calories from animal products, only 3.2 billion people would have enough food to eat. Let's suppose that figure were lowered by just 10 percent. In that case, 4.2 billion people would be sustained. That's over 1 billion people more! So just think of what the complete removal of all animal products could do. The entire world population, more than 6.3 billion people, would go to bed every night with a full stomach.

The Animals

According to FAO, more than 60 billion animals are killed every year whether for food or product consumption. This figure is absolutely staggering, and it doesn't even take into consideration the number of animals killed accidentally, whether by farm incident, losing a home to crop cultivation or for mere sport.

In Animal Liberation, author Peter Singer explains the reasoning behind animal rights. He states that the basic principle of equality does not require equal or identical treatment; it requires equal consideration. This is a sentiment shared by many vegans. The question is not whether animals can reason or speak or function at a higher learning level. An inability to state their cause doesn't mean they don't have one. The question, asserts Singer, is whether animals deserve to be free of suffering.

Other proponents of animal rights would point to the selective nature of our diet. Eating a dog would be viewed with disgust in any American home. But a pig? Not an issue. Why is that? In this instance we have two animal species – just two among thousands – that have an equal ability to feel pain, fright, frustration, and contentment. Yet even with their "equal" abilities as higher thinkers, we feel justified in considering one species worthy of our loving homes and one species worthy of being our dinner.

At one time, the term "humane meat" began to take root in the agriculture industry in hopes it would improve relations with animal rights advocates. It meant that eating meat and dairy was justified if the animals were raised in good conditions and not mistreated. That concept, never accepted by vegans, is now beginning to erode with the general population too. Increasingly, reports are published of continued animal cruelty, and secret recordings by nonprofits such as Mercy for Animals are providing the proof. When we see the evidence on video, it is much harder to forget at our next meal how the meat came to be upon our plates. It is also much easier to see the value of a vegan lifestyle beyond its health benefits.

Righting Social Injustices

The social injustice of meat, dairy, egg and honey consumption is a direct result of speciesism: the belief that being human is a valid reason for human animals to have greater rights than non-human animals. To illustrate this point, a vegan will justifiably ask: Isn't raising animals for consumption another form of slavery? Treating a living and responsive creature as an object whose sole purpose is to fulfill our needs...this is slavery in its purest form.

Gary Smith, co-founder of Evolutus, has remarked, "150 years ago, they would've thought you were absurd if you advocated for the end of slavery. 100 years ago, they would have laughed at you for suggesting that women should have the right to vote. Fifty years ago, they would've objected to the idea of African-Americans receiving equal rights under the law. Twenty-five years ago, they called you a pervert if you advocated for gay rights. They laugh at us now for suggesting that animal slavery be ended. Someday they won't be laughing."

What's most striking about this is not the list of victimized and oppressed. Mankind has suffered victimization since the beginning of its history. What's most impressive is that the groups Smith refers to were successful in achieving their goals, however far-reaching they seemed at the time. They advocated their cause with an unwavering commitment to succeed that yielded results once never dreamed possible and were rewarded with magnificent outcomes. In the case of animals, they have no voice to advocate their cause, so it is imperative that we feel compassion towards them. Vegans are the human "voice" of non-human animals. Perhaps Will Tuttle, Ph. D., author of The World Peace Diet, provided the most effective inspiration for dedicating ourselves to the vegan lifestyle when he said, "The light of the infinite spiritual source of all life shines in all creatures. By seeing and recognizing this light in others, we free both them and ourselves. This is love."

Spreading the message

As more and more information comes to light that evidences why a vegan lifestyle has such positive global ramifications, we now turn to sharing that message with others. Every time we turn on our laptop and connect to the Internet, we have the opportunity to educate others on the importance of veganism through various social media sites. We are now able to meet, support, and discuss with people from all over the world instead of being limited to our nearby communities. The Internet provides an opportunity for vegans to stand together through online petitions and fundraising too.

As convenient and effective as the Internet is, let's not forget personal, face-to-face communication. Open a dialogue with a stranger or include a stranger in a conversation you're having with a vegan. Volunteer in a vegan group whose mission is to spread the word. Great strides can be made by working together. Lead by example and model veganism for others. Many people believe they'll have to sacrifice too much of what they love if they become a vegan. Invite guests over and prepare a vegan meal to show them what the food is like, but don't stop there: send the recipes home with them if they're interested. That small effort on your part will go a long way. The small amount of time you save them in searching for a recipe might be enough to encourage them to try out a new vegan lifestyle.

It is important to share the reasons for a vegan lifestyle; it's also critical to use the right means for doing so. In *Why We Love Dogs, Eat Pigs, and*

Wear Cows, social psychologist Dr. Melanie Joy says, "Often, vegan advocates assume that a person's defensiveness is the result of selfishness or apathy, when in fact it is much more likely the result of systematic and intensive social conditioning." With this in mind, approach each person thoughtfully and carefully. Remember, you're asking people to turn their world upside down. Their scepticism is natural. A pushy, demanding, or righteous presentation of facts usually only ensures defensiveness, annoyance, and a pre-determination to not try something new. Using a compassionate, gentle approach will yield greater benefits by far.

LAYING DOWN OUR WEAPON

More than 50 years ago Mahatma Gandhi said, "The most violent weapon on earth is the table fork." Today, science is able to prove the truth in Gandhi's statement. The negative effects of consuming animal products surround us: our forests are being decimated, the climate is increasingly unstable and atrocities against animals are worsening. The good news is that it's not too late to stop the devastation. I said earlier in this chapter that the common thread binding humanity is its desire for harmony and peace.

It was also Gandhi who said, "Be the change you want to see in the world." Each and every one of us has the opportunity to be the change we want to see in the world through the choices we make. I choose to follow in Gandhi's footsteps by living a vegan lifestyle towards harmony and peace. What do you choose? Here, now, is your opportunity. It's as simple as living vegan. If we individually do our part as vegans, then collectively we will have taken massive strides toward achieving our goal for peace. Will you join me in changing the world?

To learn more about a vegan lifestyle, please visit my website at www.MrsGreenjeansPlantsSeeds.com/book, where you can get a free list of hidden animal ingredients in foods.

Break Through Your Barriers & Live Your Dreams

SANDRA WESTLAND

Every woman deserves to feel powerful and successful, and the opportunity to do so stands right before her. She doesn't have to be a warrior to smite every dragon or burn down every obstacle that stands in her way. She simply needs to connect with and be her real, authentic self. So her journey to success begins by standing still, by being curious about the world of potential that exists within her and in front of her, and by understanding her inner world in order to ignite change in her outer one towards her success.

But, what stops her from becoming the author of her own life, from being all she can be? The glass ceiling, the unofficial barrier that prevents women from rising up to executive positions or from running their successful businesses, does still exist. Yet, in my twenty-five years of education, hypno-psychotherapy and peak performance training, I see, more significantly, an individual's own inner glass ceiling capping and limiting the success in life that is there for the taking.

To be a woman is to be extraordinary. We all have it within us to move beyond an ordinary life and its everyday limitations to embrace our desires and possibilities, harness our untold natural potential and live the life we are meant to live —a life of personal freedom in which we simply are our natural, awesome selves. Your power is switched on when you embrace, embody, express and enjoy being a woman. Your energy is released when you learn to live truly in your own skin. I love being a woman, and I love continuing to find out just what that is like for me.

This is a journey of discovering your place in life as a woman and as a woman in business, a voyage into your inner mind's processing and the terrain of your inner world, deeper than your conscious mind can be aware of. It is an expedition through self-alignment, forming the detail of your desired outcomes, shaping your life to fit with your passions, sourcing the energy that drives you, thus smashing your glass ceiling and allowing your transformation to unfold. Just as I experienced my own first steps, I want you also to stride out along this path and the journey of becoming your potential. The message I write within the pages of *Smashing Your Glass Ceiling* takes you through this fascinating journey where "Wow, I didn't realize that" and "No wonder I wasn't getting to where I wanted to" are familiar insights.

HOW DOES IT ALL WORK?

The tools you will need for such a journey of self-discovery are drawn from Neuro-Linguistic Programming (NLP), guided imagery, and a gentle questing into uncovering your own uniqueness and meaning in life. In blending these time-tested methods into one programme, it's possible to break through all that's holding you back in life.

From my own personal experience as a woman and as a psychotherapist and trainer, I've found that one of the most powerful tools we naturally have and need to embrace first is the power of imagination; even if you think you have one or not, you really do have an amazing, creative imagination. It just may need awakening and a little encouraging. I would love to show you just how powerful your imagination can be and how crucial it is to connect with you and be your own woman. In beginning this imaginative journey, you are sparking off a chain of events that produce fundamental changes in your physical body, starting with the neurological processes that will link to your biology and produce within you "decision states" leading to the different outcomes that you want, easily and naturally. Imagine the decisions that you can make or the actions that you can take when you are feeling confident, in balance and aligned to your vision, compared to the choices that you opt for when you are upset, anxious, depressed and out of sync with yourself.

By guiding your imagination, you can form an internal vision in which you are taking the right path for you to succeed in your life, and then formulate just what that is. As you immerse yourself in the excitement and the thrill of being on the right road to greatness, you tap into the inner confidence and self-reliance, inner freedom and success awareness that generate your momentum to smashing your glass ceiling. The power is always within you. It's just a case of summoning and connecting with it.

Imagine also gaining new understanding into how you process information from your "now" experiences, how you view the world, how you communicate with others and how they communicate with you. Imagine how much easier your life would be. You can learn how to recognize ways of processing external data and how, by modifying your communication in a way that makes sense to others, your relationships become infinitely warmer, richer and more connected.

Think about meeting me in the flesh for the first time, already knowing how my inner world works. Wouldn't it be good to know I'm an auditory person? Why? Well, my world is very much filtered through sounds. I will be finely tuned into noise ... all noise. I will get distracted with too much of it, and I will recognize very slight changes in your voice, tone and pitch. So I will hear a hint of doubt or an emotion rising from within you just by hearing your voice. If you speak too slowly or very loudly, this will create a dissonance within me. If you use language that talks about "viewing something" or "seeing what you mean" or "having a handle on this or that" instead of "sounds like" or "listen to", I will feel a mismatch between us. Don't click your pen or tap it on the table if you want me to be relaxed! It's only a slight inner discomfort, but it undeniably shapes how I experience you and your communication. Upon our meeting, if you appreciate my world and I appreciate yours, we will hit it off with ease. I will look to communicate to you through your world, which may be visual, auditory, kinesthetic or auditory digital, all very different ways of experiencing and processing, and you can do the same for me.

GETTING TO KNOW YOUR GLASS CEILING

Your internal glass ceiling may have been created from prejudgments, prejudices, cultural and social attitudes that operate deep within the unconscious, taken in when young. So, it's crucial to find these out and know how they work for you, to understand the inner conflicts that are holding you back and what they mean. In speaking with a senior executive upon her reading *Smashing Your Glass Ceiling*, she'd suddenly become aware of how she was dressing like a man for her banking boardroom meetings. It wasn't her at all, but after further exploration, she realized she had unconsciously thought it would help men relate to her and allow her to be "taken seriously". She was shocked at how unconscious this had been, but she was relieved to learn it and is now enjoying the fun of finding out who she is as a woman in business and what clothes this exploration leads her to wearing. It is only by excavating these unconscious gender biases and other judgments that contribute towards making your own ceiling that you can reveal your real, natural self to yourself and the world. In understanding yourself more and knowing just who you are and how you are in the world, you become free to choose how to respond to situations and to people, and then you really begin to own your own life.

I am wondering just what you are thinking, having read these thousand plus words. Is this possible for you or is your glass ceiling giving you bother, preventing you from imagining and thinking of all that you can be? What does your ceiling hold and what is it whispering to you right now? What is your "default" setting?

Are you someone who assumes you won't find a car parking space and prove yourself right, or do you simply know that it doesn't matter where you park and thus usually find one just when and where you need it? Is a potential redundancy at work a chance to do something different, or a terrible catastrophe that you will never escape? Your attitudes play a massive part in your life experiences, and to how much you can grow. Zig Ziglar's famous saying "Your attitude determines your altitude" is so true. So, how do your attitudes determine how successful you can be?

I have lived and refined through my own personal journey a framework of all the things that are crucial to help you aspire to be. Let's make a start right now, something to get you thinking. Let's peek into those achieving just what you want and begin to emulate some of what they do and how they are. It's as good a place as any to start!

In NLP terms, this is called "modeling". In modeling the behaviors and habits of successful people, we're seeking to learn from successful businesswomen and successful women just what it is that they do, and what it is that they have that makes them successful; not to become them, but to incorporate their winning behaviours into our repertoire, choosing those which are congruent with us and amplifying them. I often explore other women that I admire and am drawn to. In carefully watching what they do and exploring this within my own life, in my way, I can open up to further resources that I naturally have, but have yet to connect with. In Sue Knight's' words, "If you spot it, you've got it." (NLP at Work, 2013)

Now to stoke up those neurological pathways as we vamp it up a little more and transport you forward into your own fabulous future. Familiarize yourself with the state of being successful with no glass ceiling, as if you've already accomplished that level of success, a dress rehearsal if you like. Put on the mantle of success and ask yourself how and what do you feel, how would your day evolve, what can you do now that you couldn't do before. How would others perceive you? Get your brain to make it a done deal so that it can look for it, search it out and create it. This is the self-fulfilling prophecy at its most positive, potent and powerful.

Anticipate now becoming friendly and familiar with a future you who has everything you need and want and to be able to use the guidance of that future you – the answers may very well surprise you. My future self enlightened me as to my fear of success! This helped me find my inner glass ceiling and the meaning of it all, so I could smash it and really begin to find out just what I could do and what was possible in life. I believe that to guide others you have to have lived the journey yourself, and so my own personal journey has and is this path too, encompassing where I am finding myself ... as a woman, an educator, therapist and businesswoman. This is a journey I don't ever intend to stop.

PEELING BACK THE ONION

There is so much more to explore! As humans, we've infinite depths, so exploring your inner beliefs, your values and mission is crucial for success. It's the peeling back of the onion, layer by layer (corny, I know), but I assure you that the exploration, while deep, is richly rewarding. Wouldn't you rather know what's holding you back and why you may feel frustrated with yourself? I know I would. I simply want to make the most of my time on this earth and experience it as much as possible. Life is to be lived and not simply endured and got through.

Excavate your inner beliefs, isolate the limiting ones that have held you back, and then you will easily and naturally begin to fly! Once figured out, you become empowered as you re-think and re-frame beliefs into being resourceful, productive and desirable, and turn them into second nature.

Let's go one deeper. Do you know just what it is that you value, all those things that are really important to you? Are they aligned with your life? These are your GPS, and if you're frustrated, feel trapped in the mundane of life or have unwanted physical/emotional symptoms, then value fine-tuning is needed for you to move forward in the direction that you want to go. Let's not be sidetracked by detours, road closures and an unclear destination. Being authentic and all that you are needs you to know what you value so that you're able to craft your mission for the ultimate alignment. In *Smashing Your Glass Ceiling* or my Success workshops , you will not short-change yourself here. I will journey with you, helping you along the way through a process of simple, yet profoundly powerful steps.

When you are fully aligned, there will be no holding you back. You'll meet the right person at the right time, and you'll have the right skills to achieve your goals. Everything will fall into place like a jigsaw puzzle, and you'll have "the strength, the patience, and the passion to reach for the stars", to borrow the words of a courageously inspiring woman, Harriet Tubman.

LOADING UP ON INTERNAL RESOURCES

It's not all plain sailing, and you *will* be derailed by the unexpected, but what makes someone a success is their ability to keep going, even when challenged. So, one of the final steps in the Programme is to load you up with the internal resources to get you through when things get sticky, and when, quite frankly, you wonder why you bother. NLP strategies reprogram how we react and respond to such times, making a monumental difference to how you experience your life. If you're feeling down on yourself, I will show you that you can change your physiology. If you're getting increasingly anxious about an upcoming meeting, you can change your self-talk, the inner conversation you're having with yourself, to something more upbeat, more encouraging and more positive.

Powerful NLP strategies are there for you to use at any time and in any situation. Your life will be richer and filled with more options when you are able to redirect your thinking and focus, stay resourceful in stressful situations, and generate behaviors and outcomes that are positive for you and your life.

Finally, if this chapter has inspired you to delve deeper into Smashing your Glass Ceiling, the book comes with a number of bonuses, some of which can be downloaded from my website, www.SmashingYourGlassCeiling.com for you to enjoy absolutely free. So, get started now and embrace the fact that you are an extraordinary woman.

TAKING THE FIRST STEP

All of us have to start somewhere. I did when I was thirty-four, when I found myself looking at twenty-six more years before retirement, counting the years and the days till the next school holiday. Not how I imagined my life would be.

By becoming curious, asking questions of myself and tapping into effective life-changing techniques that opened me up to the power and potential of the mind, I'm on a fascinating journey. I'm continuing to smash my own internal glass ceiling, and am living out my passion to enhance the lives of other women. I am certainly not "sorted out", nor have I "self-actualized" and not every day is "grrreat", but I know that every day is an adventure with the chance to grow further and find out more about just what is possible.

The more women I meet and work with, the more I learn and the more I gather evidence to support my belief that, as women, we owe it to ourselves to be extraordinary. This is my invitation to you to take the first steps with me on your own journey of becoming all you wish to be.

Sandra Westland is an experienced educator, therapist and successful businesswoman who helps others to find their passion and fulfil their dreams. She has a Master's degree in Existential Psychotherapy, an Education Honours degree, and is a practicing Advanced Hypnotherapist and NLP practitioner. Her doctoral thesis explores women and their relationship with their bodies. She is the author of Smash Your Glass Ceiling and co-author of Thinking Therapeutically.

Sandra is a Director of the Contemporary College of Therapeutic Studies, where she trains people at life changing junctures to be aspiring therapists, so they too can enjoy the enriching privilege of helping others to find their path in life. She is also a co-founder of Self Help School™, which provides psycho-education for the public and is an international speaker on the power of the mind for change.

Evolution of Consciousness for the Entrepreneur

Accelerate Your Consciousness, Master Your Life

AUDREE TARA WEITZMAN

"Be the change that you wish to see in the world."

– Mahatma Gandhi

"With great power comes great responsibility"

– Voltaire, Uncle Ben Spiderman

We have been through the Industrial Evolution, the Scientific Evolution and the Technological Evolution. Now is the time for the Evolution of Consciousness. A term prevalent in the personal growth and transformational communities, the Evolution of Consciousness comes out of the ever growing New Age movement. It involves the process of self-awareness and the awakening of the human mind. In truth, it is about personally understanding and awakening to our own behaviors, belief systems and the answers to two critical questions: "Does this serve me?" and "Do I want to live this way?

What does this have to do with you, the entrepreneur? Self-awareness can be a powerful tool in the development of your success.

YOUR THOUGHTS AND BEHAVIORS CREATE YOUR REALITY

We are facing a critical time in our human history. I say critical because our economy, ecology and the human race are struggling for survival. The stress of maintaining your life and excelling to a better way of living has become unbalanced in the "me" culture that we have become. This struggle for survival has an effect on a personal scale: financial hardships, loss of jobs, market crashes, housing devaluations and a lack of well being. We are living fearful lives and have lost connections to both our inner selves and the outer world around us.

You can say that this cataclysmic way of thinking has gone on for centuries. Why do we now need to become aware of our behaviors and how we live? It is because all that we have accomplished, created and discovered can now be utilized for the self-preservation of the planet and the human race. We can take what we have learned and create a way of life that supports community, growth, prosperity and the regeneration of a damaged ecology. I see the Evolution of Consciousness as a coming together of all the past evolutionary processes, and the using of our higher awareness to shift and change the way we live in the world. We can then create a world where we are living to our fullest potential.

So, how does an entrepreneur fit into this world of instability and chaos? Every entrepreneur is a visionary. You think outside the box. Your thoughts and belief systems control who you are and what you become. You are looking for a way to succeed beyond what is expected of you. At the same time, however, everyone else in your life has his or her limited thoughts and belief systems. The outside support for your great adventure (owning your own business) is, therefore, weak, or sometimes non-existent. The evolution of your consciousness and the awareness of your mind's thoughts and belief systems will be your strongest supporter on the road to success.

Human beings are automatically hardwired for failure. It is ingrained in our being that we are less than perfect. Most people live their lives with minds full of negative thoughts. Those thoughts keep telling them they are not good enough, or that they do not have the power to create an amazing life. In fact, those thoughts often say "you do not deserve to have an amazing life". On average, people walk through life sick, poor and lacking enthusiasm or joy for life. They go to school, and then work at a job that meets less than their fullest potential.

You are the exception. For you, there is one big difference in life; you have a dream to do something different. You want to make a difference or do something better than anyone else does. How are you going to accomplish your dreams and live to your fullest potential with all the obstacles knocking at your door? The secret is to evolve your consciousness.

Consciousness by definition means to be aware or have self- awareness. To evolve your consciousness is to follow a process that leads to an unfolding of your self-awareness — that is, the awareness of how you live and behave according to your thoughts and belief systems. And, the evolved consciousness of an entrepreneur is a mindset that allows you to transform yourself continuously into the most successful you. You can then live your life purpose, be in a state of well being and accomplish your heart's desire.

Imagine what it will be like when you are acting and living in your highest potential. Your business, branding, marketing, the operations of your company and your relationships —with yourself, your partners and employees, your audience and clients — will all flow in an effortless way. Imagine your life flowing in abundance, with the ability to see your visions clearly and to manifest your dreams into reality. That is what the evolution of your consciousness will do for you. That is why your Evolution of Consciousness is the most important piece of the puzzle, your greatest tool for success.

THE PROCESS OF AN EVOLVED CONSCIOUSNESS

So how do you become this evolved conscious mastermind of business and personal success? How do you evolve into your fullest potential? There is a guided process to give you the tools you need to clear out the old patterning and create an awakening. The steps are:

1. Acquiring the knowledge or belief that everything is energy.

The first step involves understanding and adopting the belief that you are made up of energy. Actually, everything is energy — a vibrational frequency of wave-like patterns that make up our universe. Energy is an electromagnetic charge that is within and surrounds your body Material objects are slow moving vibrational frequencies (energy) that make up matter. Thoughts are fast moving vibrational frequencies that are invisible to the naked eye, but still move and create our reality. This concept is sometimes abstract, but there is a lot of information to research at your leisure. You may want to read about The Law of Attraction or about manifesting your visions into reality. You might also watch the movie "The Secret".

As an entrepreneur, your greatest tool will be your knowledge of energy and how to manage it to master your life, your relationships and your business. Energy affects how we are in relationship to ourselves and others. It impacts how we feel on a daily basis and how our vision of life's purpose or our business is projected and manifested into the world.

For example, there are some people who, for no reason, you just cannot seem to like. They are very negative, and you feel drained when you see them. Then, there are other people who you love to be around because they are happy, have a glow about them and are especially positive. You might say it's about how they act or behave, but it is really about the energy that they put out into the world. The same goes for your business. If you know about energy you can shift the energies in your life to attract the clients you want.

Importantly, your energy moves based on your thought process. That is why they say if you have negative thoughts you will get sick. This is true. Your thoughts create energy. In an instant, you can shift your negative thoughts to positive ones. And in turn you can change your negative energy into positive energy. In sum, "*Energy goes where consciousness flows*".

Energy is an inherent tool at your disposal; a tool that, if you choose not to use, will be there anyway, reacting to your subconscious mind, an event, which you do not want to happen in your life.

2. Grounding your energy so that you become a stable force of energy.

Life is chaos. Constantly shifting, moving and changing. There is no way to predict or control what happens in your life. This is the cause of all stress, anxiety and grief. I see life, especially during times of transformation, as a tornado swirling around you. It becomes very difficult to deal with things or to make the proper decisions (or even function, for that matter) when life is coming at you like a storm. The drama of life picks you up and lands you in any place, usually on the top of your head. And, for an entrepreneur, this tornado takes on speed and velocity, tenfold. Flying by the seat of your pants is an understatement.

If you are not careful, the decision-making process can mean life or death for your business, your dreams, your life purpose and your financial stability. Grounding your energy will allow you to be calm and stable while the chaos of life is swirling about you. You can become the calm in the center of the storm. In this calm place, you are able to see the whole picture of what is in front of you, and you will no longer be held hostage by emotional reactions to any drama. There is a centered feeling within you, and that is when you will be most effective.

In my training as a healer, I have found that grounding meditation is the foundation for any energy/healing work. You cannot be effective at moving energy if you are not grounded. You cannot make important life altering or business altering decisions if you are not grounded.

To make stable calm decisions, your energy needs to be in your body. I know that sounds a bit strange but, as humans, we have the habit of moving our energies up and outside of our physical bodies. We are not even aware of what we are doing. The energy leaves the physical body because of the emotional pain and suffering that we experience from life; it is easier to cope when we do not feel the pain.

When the energetic body is not connected to the physical form, it causes the body to feel anxious. It can cause a sense of being out of control, unsafe. This experience may cause physical symptoms like heart palpitations and other unproductive side effects. Think about a balloon on a string that is not connected to anything else. The balloon floats away. That is your energy and your consciousness floating away and, with it, the ability to function effectively.

Actually, it is extremely important to ground your energy into the earth itself. Some people have done yoga or used other techniques, such as guided meditation, and imagined roots growing from their feet into the ground. These techniques are based on centuries old teachings that say to anchor your body energy into the earth about three to four feet. There is real science behind these practices. There are electromagnetic grids in the earth's surface, and we connect the energy body into the earth's electromagnetic grids. This gives us a sense of security, belonging and calm.

In 2004, while doing my grounding techniques for meditation and healing work, I discovered a relatively new technique. I was forced to go deeper into the earth to ground my energy. I felt the connection of my energy field anchoring into something very powerful. What I have since learned is that I was anchoring into a permanent electromagnetic field of the earth. Although there is no science as of yet to validate what I was doing, through time and experience I have found this to be a very powerful grounding technique. I have taught it to many of my clients, some with stage four cancers, some facing terminal illnesses (they are in various places of instability).

I also have used this technique with my clients going through life transitions and major upheavals, as well as with those needing to feel safe and calm before making important life decisions. My clients who have used this grounding technique instantaneously felt an improved state of being. There is no waiting; the improved state of being happens as soon as you do the technique.

And, with practice, this technique becomes so easy that it is requires just a quick thought to become grounded; your consciousness and your physical body are calm, centered and balanced in a way that makes you feel safe and unaffected by what is happening around you. You will then begin to live and function through non-emotional reactions to the chaos and drama of life. This will be a great tool in your daily functioning. And, it can determine your success rate in making important business and life decisions.

To learn about this technique and how to use it on your own, please visit **(evolve2b.com...password: onlyone).**

3. Using energy to clear your negative thoughts and belief systems.

The entrepreneur is a master visionary. The spark of his or her thoughts and the dreams that they build, lead to the creation of a product or business, to fill the needs of the many. Entrepreneurs go against society's grain and the protests of the subconscious mind. Then there is the ego; everyone is watching you, secretly wanting you to fail. Or your own self-sabotage tries to take you down — not to mention how nerve-wracking it can be to make all the correct decisions about branding and marketing yourself and your business.

As an entrepreneur, your mindset must be clear and clean of any negative thoughts. Since thoughts are energy, they can literally reach out and affect your relationship with the outside world. It is, therefore, imperative that you erase any negative thoughts from your mind. Being successful is based on how well you manage and clear your thoughts, your consciousness and your energy.

So, what are negative thoughts? They are the ones that speak to you in your mind and judge everything that you do. Sometimes they are things your parents have told you, or they are based on experiences you had in the past. Some thoughts are from you, telling yourself you are not worthy, good enough, smart enough, do not have any money; the list goes on.

Then there are thoughts of your own greatness, how amazing you are and how no one can beat you or your product. Those thoughts will get you in trouble too; in business a thought can keep you from paying attention to improving your products or services.

In sum, thoughts are your ego, and your ego is a manifestation of an untruth. It is how you perceive yourself and the world based on past experiences. The ego makes up stories for us to believe and cuts us off from having an experience based in the present moment. It is the ego that will destroy your hopes and dreams. This is not ego bashing; the ego has long served you and has been a great asset in so many ways. But it has been running the "show" for your whole life. Now, to reach your fullest potential and the best life or business you can create, your ego needs to take a step back. At **evolve2b.com,** I give you a tool to clear your negative mind set gracefully, quickly and easily.

The process of the Evolution of Consciousness is the empowerment of you taking responsibility for your life. You become the master of your reality and create the life or business that you desire. When you are aware of your negative thoughts and behavior patterns, and you make the decision to let them go, you move into a place of positive thoughts, and begin to manifest a very powerful reality for yourself. This reality is filled with a presence of your own truth, living in the moment and knowing that you have the ability and tools to have what you desire.

4. Manifesting your desires from the heart.

The concept of manifesting your desires (or creating your reality) is something that has been much talked about in the past few years. When the movie, "The Secret," came out, it introduced the idea that it is possible to have the life you desire by asking for it. In fact, "The Secret" became the most popular source of information on manifesting and The Law of Attraction. What the movie doesn't mention is that this information about manifesting your desire, is based in an old paradigm (knowledge) used in a time when the earth vibrated at a different energetic frequency. There is a science to it, which you can read about in detail in my book, *Body Of Light, the Evolution of Consciousness Through the New Chakra System*.

The crucial point coming out of that science is that something about The Law of Attraction has changed and, so, the technique for manifesting has changed. Now, energy is very fast moving, and that changes the way we relate to ourselves and each other. We are coming into the world of peace; we are shifting into an era of living in our hearts. Why is that important for manifestation?

The old way to manifest was to have a vision which would shift your thoughts and move the energy to create your desires. Easy, right? It works, but is problematic in that, often, along with the thought of what you wanted, came a thought of how it might be impossible or that you are unworthy, In that case, the negative thought canceled out the vision.

The solution in this new energy is not to have a vision. Instead, go deeper, out of your mind (where the vision is) and into your heart, where your desire is. Yes, the heart is where manifestation takes place in this new era! For a great tool to teach you how to manifest from the heart and experience manifestation in this higher vibrational energy, please go to **(evolve2b.com).**

To create and manifest what you desire into reality, it must be done from the heart. There can be no attachment to how it manifests. There is no business plan for manifestation. That is not The Law of Attraction. The Law of Attraction says like energies (thoughts move energy) attract to each other and what you desire will manifest. The most powerful energetic wave patterns are in the heart.

... the heart is far more than a simple pump ... (it is) a highly complex, self-organized information processing center with its own functional "brain" that communicates with and influences the cranial brain... These influences profoundly affect brain function and most of the body's major organs, and ultimately determine the quality of life." — **The Institute of HeartMath**

If you are going into business to create destruction or greed, the techniques I've been talking about are not for you; it won't work. Those negative emotions are low vibrational frequencies and thought forms and will no longer be tolerated in this new paradigm. However, If you are envisioning a business product or service to help make the world a better place because you know that you can improve on a system, or want to make a difference in the world and in your life, then this knowledge will work. These tools can only be used for the highest good of man.

Remember that the mind is not a perfected state of being where there are no negative thoughts. You must drop all of your vision into your heart. Breathe in your business plan — not the step-by-step process, but the end result of your goals and vision. Feel what it is like to have your successful business, all the support that you need and beyond what you can imagine. Expect that you will have the life of your dreams, feel what it's like to live in that place of complete happiness and then let it go. When negative thoughts come into your mind, use the tools I gave you to release them.

5. Stepping into the new paradigm of business and living your highest potential.

Once you have learned this process of understanding and harnessing your body energies for good, you will be able to create and manifest the business of your dreams — no, more than that — a business beyond your wildest dreams. This is especially true for entrepreneurs because coming from an evolved consciousness means that you will:

- Maintain calm and balance to make important decisions
- Clear your limiting negative thoughts and belief systems
- Living your fullest potential, vibrant and healthy — physically mentally emotional and spiritually
- Be able to manifest your desires quickly and easily

Nothing in your business, or your life, will ever be the same.

Audree Weitzman uses her knowledge and skill as a healer, reads the Akashic Records and incorporates her training in energy based life coaching into a formula she developed called Intuitive Strategies Coaching, please go to WWW.EVOLVE2B.COM for more information

How To Gain Abundant Wealth

KAY EVE

This advice is aimed at two groups of people – first, those who heard the name of God but have not taken further action and second, those from a practising Christian background who have lapsed.

If, however, you are an atheist then the teachings described here cannot help you. I wish it were otherwise, but I cannot change how the universe is. Without belief, you cannot have God's spiritual help in your search for wealth and wellbeing. Without belief, you must rely on only human knowledge to see you through the difficult times.

The issue is that Christian teachings are haunted by two very wrong ideas. Firstly, the notion that suffering is good for you and that we must each "bear our own cross". One such example is that Mother Theresa of Calcutta refused medicine to patients in her "hospitals" because of the belief that suffering was "good for the soul." This was not the Middle Ages, but only 20 years ago, showing how deeply embedded the idea that "suffering is good, yet pleasure is dangerous" still is within Christianity even to this day. I won't deal with this idea here extensively other than to say that there are many churches that will tell you the good news, that God wants us to be happy – and what's wrong with being happy? I advise you to visit an evangelical church. The worst that can happen is you'll have a good laugh.

The second wrong impression within Christianity is that it is wrong to long for material gains. Jesus famously overturned money changers' tables in the Temple. He said "it is easier for a camel to go through the eye of a needle than for someone who is rich to enter the kingdom of God". I hope to show that what God hates isn't making money, but acquiring it dishonestly or hoarding it all to yourself. Instead, Christian teaching encourages us to live a comfortable life with your loved ones and to do good with the excess. This interpretation is often ridiculed as "praying for money", particularly by spiritual people who I want to reach. Good people also deserve to succeed! So I ask you to keep an open mind, and to give me benefit of a doubt and give careful consideration to what I have to say.

I'm certainly not saying that the Bible tells you that if you ask for gifts from God then they will just fall into your lap! Many of the good things that Gods gives us are quite unasked for – sometimes things will just come miraculously. However, what the teachings say is that if you ask, He will help you to help yourself. You will have to supply the hard work for financial success or personal happiness, but God will be right by your side.

Read on and discover God's love for us all. I know in my heart that if we start looking closely, we can find messages of encouragement that God gives mankind, messages that have mostly been covered over or shunned. I'm here to try and bring out the truth, that God wants us to know His desire for everyone to be happy and have a meaningful, fulfilling life.

And so, I thank God every day for everything that was created directly by Him and indirectly by humans in our world. I am so grateful to be here amongst all of you today.

THE GREAT DISCOVERY

When we think of our galaxy, we know that it is shaped just like a fried egg with the yellow yolk in the middle and a disc of white surrounding it. In the outer edge of the disc is our sun, with one of its planets that we call Earth, which is found to be a safe place for all living things.

During the 19th and 20th centuries, scientists gradually discovered how the universe and the earth formed and evolved. The human race had already been running around planet earth for thousands of years, living and breeding on the planet quite successfully when at peace but killing each other in times of war. Those ancient people had no knowledge of how the earth was formed, but still some of them knew the wealth teachings, and so they came to be wealthy and successful.

If you look at the world's religions today, the only faiths that teach us how to live with Abundant Wealth are the teaching of the Torah for Jews and the Old and New Testaments for Christians. The Abundant Wealth teachings were recorded in all the books we call the Bible, within which one can acquire the keys to unlock wealth and happiness.

More and more people are now searching for words of guidance from the sages of old and from modern businessmen and businesswomen alike. One may not realise that the roots of the valuable teaching from modern day "coaches" actually originate from Christian doctrine. Most people in our modern world do not know how to use and apply the keys successfully to their own lives. But through keeping in mind these teachings and keys, it is possible to achieve your goals and attain wealth, success, happiness and wellbeing.

The only thing that can maintain an abundance of wealth, success and prosperity is God. He has played the biggest part in all our lives whether we realise it or not. People can say they don't believe in God, but if they do, they won't have access to His teachings for success. A lot of people believe in other religions, but abundance only comes down to us from the most powerful, the most almighty, the most gracious and the most merciful one called God. The truth is that there is only one key in the universe and God himself has the key. By praising and asking God for His Abundant Wealth's codes you will learn how to apply the codes for yourself and become successful in every aspect of your life.

The simple question is how to become wealthy? If you believe in God, you will discover these Abundant Wealth's codes and be able to use these codes to unlock for yourself whatever your heart desires, in your personal life, business, work or family. When you have learned this, you will have learned the secret of one of the most satisfying experiences of life. You may say "Well, that's okay for those who already know God, but what about people that do not know or have never heard of God before?"

If you happen to be later, that is ok; it is very easy to join this group of enlightened. By way of illustration, I will call it a club. As you already know, if you aren't a member of a certain club, you cannot receive the access, knowledge or privileges which members can. To be in God's presence is like being in God's club just like the other Christian or religious sects' clubs.

With God we have free will to choose to worship Him or not. That is your personal choice. God does not need anything from you except to receive your sincere love and your worship. God does not want you to sacrifice anything to

Him. He has already sacrificed his own beloved son Jesus Christ for us over two thousand years ago.

Firstly, you need to believe that there is such a thing as the Supreme Being who is commonly referred to as "God", with His own special holy names by which He would prefer to be called. Without this belief, you will not have your wealth key's codes to work. If you do not believe that God exists, then why in the universe or on earth would you expect any of His Abundant Wealth's codes to work for you?

Secondly, endeavour to believe that God has the power to grant you your Wealth codes to unlock the doors of the universe and give you all aspects of success and abundant wealth. God can indeed be reached directly, for there is no distance between Him and His Son.

If you are not in God's club you are an outsider, you will not receive full wisdom to understand all of God's instructions laid out before your eyes. As Jesus has told his disciples in Mark's Gospel,

Mark 4:12 Jesus said, *"When they see what I do, they will learn nothing. When they hear what I say, they will not understand. Otherwise, they will turn to me and be forgiven."*

The "forgiven" word here means to be freed from wrong decisions, wrong choices, etc. So your faith in Jesus will make these mysterious passages, the codes, clear.

EVERYTHING IS POSSIBLE

First you need to do everything physically and mentally possible to make a good connection with God!

When we discover that we are known and understood by God, it can be a very profound and moving experience. Sometimes your spouse or best friend may know or understand you on the surface, but deep down you may feel like you are alone. And yet no matter how well you are known or understood by others, no one can understand you better than God himself. As King David has put it;

Psalm 139:1-4 NIV
"O Lord, you have searched me and you know me. You know when I sit and when I rise; you perceive my thoughts from afar. You discern my going out and my lying down; you are familiar with all my ways. Before a word is on my tongue; you know it completely. O Lord."

If you believe that God exists in the world like the ancient people of past times did, then you will want to worship the Almighty for the successes in your life. But how can you actually get a real and intimate connection to Him? The sincerity of your heart is the key to success.

Three steps to Calmness:

1. Find solitude with God, away from other people and distractions. By shutting out the sights and sounds around, you will make it easy to tune in with God.

2. Find a comfortable position, select a chair or a corner of your bed. Go to the same place at the same time in the same position every day. Consistency is of the utmost importance.

3. Before you begin, relax and take a few deep breaths. Let your mind be quiet and your body relaxed. When your mind quietens, you may know the conscious presence of God that says "Be still and know that I am God." Psalm 46:10

Now you are ready to start making a connection.

Three Steps to Listening:

1. The first step of prayer is to praise God, such as by citing the Lord's Prayer as in Matthew 6: 9-13. Let your prayer begin by praising God and you will soon find yourself in a frame of mind with Him.

2. Let some positive thinking and praying enter your mind. The secret of success is thinking and believing positively, and the same is true in prayer.

3. Ask Him to speak to you and tell Him about the things that matter to you. Whatever problems or difficulties you have, you can rely on Him for comfort, stability and the material things that the world has to offer. Once you have things off your chest, remain quite still and relaxed and listen!

By modern standards in the developed world, very few of us are really suffering. The atheists down the street will probably have all they need and live physically as well as you, perhaps even a little better. Yet, if you ask God, you will receive more blessings than they ever will and be in a better place with a better quality of life, with all the things you ask for that can be truly beneficial to you.

EXPECTING THE UNEXPECTED

Secondly you must believe that he has the power to help us and wants to help us all!

When you have asked God for the things I have described above, one final step remains - the "receiving in advance", or the assurance that your prayer will be answered. You need to thank Him and to strongly assert your confidence that He is going to provide the answer to your request. Filling your heart with positive thoughts will help to ensure that God will allow these things to happen.

Yet, how can you be assured that a constant relationship with God will produce answered prayer? The answer lies within the Abundant Wealth codes, within the heart of answered prayer, and within the following everyday Bible verses, such as;

Matthew 17:20
If you have faith as a grain of mustard seed, you shall say unto this mountain, "Remove from here" and it will move. Nothing will be impossible for you." (The "mountain" in this parable of Jesus means one of our life's great crises.)

Matthew 21:22
If you believe, you will receive whatever you ask for in prayer.

Mark 21:24
Therefore, I tell you whatever you ask for in prayer, believe that you have received it and it will be yours.

However, do not mix up the word "Faith" with "Belief". To believe that God can answer and is able to deliver all of the things being asked for in prayer, this is not faith. Everyone can have faith. The prayer of faith means trusting in God to do something but truly believing in God means to know that God is honest and will do what He says He will. It is to believe unhesitatingly that He is on the verge of doing it and that even now, the answer is on the way to you.

Many people also misconceive faith as desire, but this is false. Many people want success, but longing, wanting and desiring success is not faith. Desire, rightly directed, can produce faith and may lead you to faith, but in itself it is not faith. When you have known God intimately, you may experience a genuine re-dedication of your heart, only to be disappointed that your prayer went unanswered. This is because God may judge that the "good" thing was not what you really need at that time. He will give you something else that's good, something that benefits your life.

Faith is a common commodity. Everyone has faith. Atheists have faith that there is no God. Animals and pets have faith in their masters. Children have faith in their parents and we have faith in our Governments to watch over our nation. It is only faith in God through truly believing in Him that will reward you with your heart's desire. As James says in James 1:6-8;.

"But when you ask God, you must believe and not doubt, because he who doubts (unbelief) is like a wave of the sea, blown and tossed by the wind. That man should not think he will receive anything from the Lord, he is a double-minded man, unstable in all he does."

Believing is an act of total trust in God; it doesn't require information, knowledge or certainty – only the free and joyful surrender in His goodness. To help with this, look for the "invisible" gifts of God. They are clearly seen in the many good things that have already happened, things that are usually taken for granted. However, God alone will not change the course of some worldly events. For instance, He doesn't interfere with situations in which people have created chaos around themselves. They must deal with the consequences of their own actions. God is very constant, but for victims caught in the chaos He will turn things around for those who have the absolute trust in Him.

Each code of Abundant Wealth is laid out in the Bible for anyone to read. It has rarely been used before because few pay attention or even try to find out the meaning that God has given freely to everyone. Established religions tell people that praying for money or success is the sin of "avarice", yet churches get rich while their congregations are told to be content with what they have. But who can build a hospital or invent a new medicine without money? It is not the money that is inherently bad; it is the people that do bad things with or for it.

Most modern day sages who have written books about God's wealth codes have hidden the source of these gifts, saying that they come from the universe instead of from God Himself. One can ask for wealth, success, love and happiness until your tongue hangs out, but you will not receive the answer without asking only God himself.

Asking others who pretend to be God for favours will end in disastrous results for you, even if it may appear to be beneficial at first. Many rich and famous people have made deals with others but there is a steep price that must be paid for this false hope. Through Jesus Christ, we have paid already and there is nothing to fear when asking for success, as long as it is done without wickedness or dishonesty.

If you are still skeptical about the wealth key's code then it will not work for you. I wish you good health and happiness, but if you remain doubtful you might as well throw this book away! To have everything that you need and desire you must make a total surrender of your heart, your love and your belief to God, the powerful and the almighty who has created this world and the universe. As is said in Hebrews 11:1-6;

"Now faith is being sure of what we hope for and certain of what we do not see …. By faith we understand that the universe was formed at God's command, so that what is seen was not made out of what was visible …. And without faith it is impossible to please God, because anyone who comes to him must believe that he exists and that he rewards (Abundant Wealth to) those who earnestly seek him."

THE TRUTH REVEALED

Who is "God" and what's wrong with the idea of a general "Supreme Being"?

God defines Himself as the great lover of mankind, and many Bible verses reveal the depth of this love.

Jeremiah 9:24
"I am the Lord, I show unfailing love, I do justice and right upon the earth; for on this I have set my heart"

Jeremiah 31:3
"I have loved you with an everlasting love; I have drawn you with loving kindness."

Mark 11:29-33
"A new command I give you: Love one another. As I have loved you, so you must love one another."

Most religious texts, Hebrew and Muslim alike, give many names of God in their own Language - seventy-two in Hebrew and up to ninety-nine for Muslims. The only one that God told Moses directly is found in Exodus 33:19. "I will call out my name, Yahweh" ("The Lord"). Even so, there are many other names given to God which reflect the compassion, kindness and generosity He had for different peoples, such as;

Yahweh-Jireh Lord will provide

Yahweh-Rohi Lord is my shepherd

Yahweh-El Shadia Lord Almighty

Yahweh-Shalom Lord of peace

Yahweh-Rapha Lord of healing

Yahweh-El-Olam	Lord everlasting
Yahweh-M'kaddesh	Lord who sanctifies

As mentioned in the Old Testament, no one can see God face-to-face and live to tell, due to his vast and glorious power being too much for our bodies of mere flesh and bone. For this reason, when God appeared to Moses He covered Moses' body with the shadow of His hand.

Exodus 33:19
"I will make all my goodness pass by before you. For I will show mercy to anyone I choose, and I will show compassion to anyone I choose."

Exodus 33:20
"but you may not look directly at my face, for no one may see me and live."

As we know from the Bible, God created the universe, the world and all living things on it. Among these creations was the Sun, which produced the light and heat that God commanded to shine upon the Earth as God had wanted from the beginning.

Genesis 1:1 & 31
"In the beginning God created the heavens and earth…And God said "let there be light."

And so, humans were born on Earth in multitudes, and from them God selected the nation of Israel and the Jewish people to work with Him. Much of the Old Testament tells of God's love towards this nation. Yet men were disobedient and uncaring towards God, turning away to worship frightful and false gods instead. And so the New Testament tells us that God sent his son, Jesus Christ, to be born as a human among us and so that we would love and worship him again. As the Bible says, if we accept that Jesus is our Lord and the son of God, then we become God's adopted children and have the right to call him Father and to ask for his Wealth Keys.

Matthew 7:11

Jesus says, "Ask and it will be given to you; seek and you will find; knock and the door will be opened to you.....which of you, if your children ask for bread, will give them a stone.....if you, then, though you are evil, know how to give good gifts to your children, how much more will your Father in heaven give good gifts to those who ask Him."

So what do we know about God so far? We know we can ask Him for help in all matter of things and that nothing is too big or small for Him to handle. We can ask Him for guidance in all of our problems because He truly cares, and we can also ask him for whatever we desire and it shall be done for us. If we know God intimately and are not happy with our present situation, then we can always ask Him to change it for the better. We must remember that there is no god other than Yahweh-God who proved his love for us by laying down his own son's life for our benefit. The people who get their prayers answered are just simple people like you and I. We must never doubt in Him and we must always rest assured; God is real. He was, He is and He will be in everyone's life.

THE ASKING

But how can you actually go about asking God for Abundant Wealth?

Everything is possible with God for those who love Him. You can trust in God that all that you ask will be fulfilled before you draw your last breath on earth, no matter how long it takes. An example can be seen in Luke Ch. 2 where Simon, the old Jewish prophet who was full of devotion to God, asked that he might meet the Messiah in his own lifetime. God answered his wishes and promised Simon would meet him before he died.

Luke 2:27-29

Led by the spirit, Simon went into the Temple. So when Mary and Joseph came to present the baby Jesus to The Lord as the law required. Simon took the baby Jesus into his arms and praised God, saying "Master, now you are dismissing your servant in peace according to your promise."

It is God's will that his children will possess Abundant Wealth and all that they desire. And so we now need to concentrate on how to build a relationship with God in order to receive his true blessings. Like any relationship, one has to dedicate oneself to make it happen. Though it is common knowledge that true human relationships are not always easy to maintain, it is different with God for he loved you first. He longed for you to love Him back, and it is up to you now to do your part.

There are only a minority of people who have a true belief in God's love and will see a miracle happen to them in their lives. It is hard for most people to love and believe in God, especially being surrounded by modern technology where things must be seen, heard, touched, felt or sensed in order to be real. God and belief in Him have become almost a myth, but the key to finding true belief is to discern God's love in your own life, which can be done in Five Steps.

1. Ask God to step into your heart and reveal his truth to you. You can do this anywhere or any time as long as it feel right to you. Once you have accepted God and Jesus into your heart, you will become an adopted child of God and you can begin building the relationship.

Revelation 3:20

Jesus says; "Look! I stand at the door and knock. If you hear my voice and open the door, I will come in, and we will share a meal together as friends."

2. Begin worshiping and praising God, whether out loud or silently in your mind. Concentrate on God's love towards your every being. Ask God to clean not only your heart, but your mind, your soul and your entire being. You must create the purest atmosphere to get positive reception of God's intuition and that small voice that speaks directly into your heart.

Nahum 1:7
"The Lord is good, a refuge in times of trouble. He cares for those who trust in him."

3. Study God's word within the Old and New Testaments, asking God for the wisdom to discern the Bible's lessons. The parables are not easily understood the first time they are read, so you must ask for God's help in deciphering them. Only then may you apply them to your personal and professional life, as generations of God's children have done before you.

Mark 4:9-12
"Anyone with ears to hear should listen and understand" … "You are permitted to understand the secret of the Kingdom of God. But I use parables *for everything I say to outsiders, so that the Scriptures might be fulfilled."*

Understand that things which you ask God for can come quickly or slowly depending on how ready you are to receive them. God knows that if he gives them to you when you are not ready, you will lose these gifts or become unable to cope with it. In time, if we use His words and apply them to our lives, we are sure to receive everything that we need or want and we may continue to ask for more.

4. Have faith that God will deliver. You can see how often many people gave up on asking things from God because they could not see any results

coming out of their prayers. Most people have forgotten what the most important part of the prayer is. They forgot to get the most authoritative person to support and speed their request so that it was heard quickly by God. Much like in a court case where you need a proper barrister to work with you to ensure the judge will rule in your favour, it is the same with God. You need your spiritual brother Jesus Christ to help with your prayers so that the Heavenly Father may execute your request. Always ask God for your needs in Jesus' name. But remember, only God knows when the time is right for you to receive his gifts, much like a doctor who knows when to give treatment to his patient. Once you understand all of the above, you can use the Bible Keys and apply them to your personal life.

Isaiah 55:11

God says; "It is the same as my word. I send it out and it always produces fruit. It will accomplish all I want it to, and it will prosper everywhere I send it."

5. Finally, you must give thanks. After you have given your prayer request, you must thank God with all your heart. The more you thank Him, the quicker his blessings will come to you. You must now concentrate on believing one hundred percent in your heart that your request is now heard by God.

There is a final condition that you need to make it work. You must understand that if you have received God's answer to your request, you will now need to get to work on the request you made. You will not receive any kind of blessing that you have not earned, much like the old wives' tale of "help yourself first and God will help you."

Proverbs 10:4

"Lazy hands make a man poor, but diligent hands bring wealth."

Proverbs 22:29

"Be sure you know the condition of your flocks, give careful attention to your herds."

The above five conditions are absolute must-dos if you want your prayer to be answered and to succeed in having God bless you with wellbeing, happiness and success in your life.

Roman 10:11

"As the Scripture says. Anyone who trusts in Him will never be put to shame."

GRATITUDE

Giving thanks is of vital importance, but just Giving to others is also important!

How well do we know the meaning of the word "gratitude"? If you want Abundant Wealth from God, you must be able to change your attitude and behaviour towards what you have been given already.

1 Timothy 6:17

"..... Their trust should be in God, who richly gives us all we need for our enjoyment. Tell them to use their money to do good. They should be rich in good works and generous to those in need. By doing this they will be storing up their treasure as a good foundation for the future so that they may experience true life."

You already know how to trust in God for the things you have asked for. Now you need to know how to act while you are waiting for God to bestow upon you the things you desire. Even if you do not have much, you still need to appreciate what you do have, that which has sustained you until now. You may hate your menial job or be in a boring business, but you must not condemn it. After all, it has kept you afloat until now.

The Key to this is that now you know how to turn things around. While appreciating what sustained you, from its original roots, God will bless it and turn it into a good thing.

Matthew 25:29

Jesus says; "For everyone who has will be given more, and they will have abundance. Whoever does not have, even what they have will be taken from them."

This first sentence above means that your need to be grateful for all the things you currently possess. This appreciation will make them become more important, even if right now they seem worthless to you. The second sentence does not mean that God will take your things away, only that without your appreciate of them, the few resources you have tend to be squandered.

In the physical realm, you may be in a job that you hate but are desperate to leave. You may want God to answer your prayers and to help you out of this predicament. In this instance, while you wait for God to manifest things that you have prayed for, you must learn to imitate God's spiritual realm in order to turn it into your real world.

Romans 8:24

".... But hope that is seen is no hope at all. Who hopes for what he already has? But we hope for what we do not yet have, we wait for it patiently."

If you know the mind of Jesus Christ, you will know that when He was in human form, everything was beautiful and perfect in God's eyes. Jesus was without worry and he was on Earth solely for the purpose of doing God's work. Nothing could harm or touch him because God's power was within him. When he was laid on the cross of crucifixion, it was because Jesus allowed himself to be, in order to fulfill the scriptures and be sacrificed as a lamb of God for all of us.

Therefore, you must have gratitude for Christ's gift because he paid with his life for your sins. You can be free of anxiety, stress, worry, distress and ill health because Jesus removed all those bad things from you. All hardships are of the physical realm; you can be free of these struggles by switching yourself to the spiritual realm.

When you know that God is by your side, your mind will be sharp and focused. No matter what sort of negative thoughts arise, you must not listen to them. They're trying to lure you away from God and all the good things that he has in store for you.

According to Christian teachings, two cosmic broadcast stations – the Light and the Dark – send signals to our brain. Any thought that is loud and clear, which urges you to react to a situation, without a proper plan, that is the enemy – the Dark. But if the thought is barely audible, if it is a soft voice emanating from the recesses of our mind, it is the song of the Light. If you are greeted with a sudden flash of intuition or inspiration, you can be certain it is from the spiritual realm.

The key to taking control of your life is to ignore the loud noise in your head and to take time to concentrate on the small, quiet sounds from God to guide you. When you succeed in blocking out the negative thoughts that manifest themselves as our greedy and selfish egos, the Light signal and all the good thoughts that come along with it are free to fill our minds. The best ideas can come forth at once and without hindrance, and you can see the way to wisdom.

In the Old Testament, during the time that king Ahab ruled in Israel, Ahab did not worship God. He killed all of God's prophets except one, Elijah. Elijah was afraid and asked for God's help. He went into a cave where he spent the night praying and waiting for God's instruction.

1 Kings 11:13

"Go out and stand before me on the mountain" the Lord told him. And as Elijah stood there, the Lord passed by, and a mighty windstorm hit the mountain. It was such a terrible blast that the rocks were torn loose, but the Lord was not in the wind. After the wind there was an earthquake, but the Lord was not in the earthquake. And after the earthquake there was a fire, but the Lord was not in the fire. And after the fire there was the sound of a gentle whisper. .... And the voice said "What are you (still) doing here, Elijah?"

Thus we can know that the gentle, whispering voice is from God, not the enemy.

You now have all the Abundant Wealth Keys in your hands, and can begin to apply them to all aspects of your life. You can begin to see success in all areas, from your personal and family life, to your professional and business life, and to your community as well.

Finally, remember this. If you care for other human beings like God cares for you, you will continue to receive God's blessing. You will please God if you lend Him a hand, doing charitable work for those less fortunate than you in this world that God has made for us all.

Profit for the Automotive Service Industry

7 Steps to Double Your Income by Improving Service

DALE F. JOHNSON

STEP 1 - INCREASE YOUR PROFIT

I can't tell you how many shop owners and service men believe that it's wrong to make "too much profit" from their work. I know it sounds counter intuitive—heck it sounds downright crazy, but I'm here to tell you it's true. I'm also here to teach the contrary, that profit is a fine thing, not only in business, but in life as well. That's why I'm going to show you how to change.

First and foremost: what is a realistic profit to expect in any aspect of business? 2%, 5%, 10%, 20%, 40%? Do you know? It's 20%. If you have a shop rate of $100, when all is said and done, a minimum of $20 of every hour billed had better be yours or you've made some serious mistakes in building your business. The same goes for the products you sell. Everyone knows that retailers take a minimum 40% mark-up on anything they sell, but did you know that sometimes a 200% mark-up is necessary? You see, the most important thing you can remember is at the end of the day you should retain a minimum profit of 20% of everything sold or serviced. Why do I say a minimum of 20%? Because if you need more in order to reach the lifestyle you want, then you should increase the profit as required. Forget anything else you've heard. You deserve this, and it can be done. Even in your own life—you should be able to take about 20% of your time each day just for you.

How do you do it? In the end it comes down to two things: how well your business model works and how well you serve your customers. From a business perspective, you need to draw an intricate model of your business while asking a series of questions: Can this part of my business earn more profit? How? Conversely, am I losing money here? If so, what do I do to fix it? What can I do to create maximum efficiency while also earning maximum profit? From a customer service perspective you need to ask: How can I do more for the customer without increasing costs? What is the maximum shop rate and parts rates that I can charge before my customer stops thinking he or she is getting full value for their dollar? They've got to believe that what you charge them is a bargain in the end. And the only way to do that is to sit down and write out every need you require fulfilled when you go to a garage yourself. This is what you must provide to each and every customer you have. And it's why you must reconstruct your business from the ground up. Where does your business, as a machine with well-oiled parts, break down? Where are you bleeding money? What are you going to do to fix these things? How can you minimize the amount of money that goes into your business and then maximize the money that comes back out? (More on this later.)

I'm going to ask you two very simple questions, and I want you to answer them honestly. When you go to work are you passionate about it? Is it what you want? If you falter in either answer, how can you work to enjoy life? After all, that is why you are in business today. You want more than a simple pay cheque. You want fulfilment. You want to be more than the masses. When you embrace the concept of work to enjoy life it doesn't mean that even if you hate your job you'll enjoy life. It means you have to love your job and then you can work to enjoy your life. And this attitude needs to encompass every hour of every living day. You must love life or, more importantly, you must love your life! You started your business to be able to enjoy the very life you are in, not my life or that of anyone else you know.

I want to show you that, by taking a few simple steps (like increasing your profit) and sticking to them, that your work will help you to enjoy the rest of your life! You'll be amazed at the transformation that will follow. So remember this: if it's a job, that's all that gets done; if it's a passion, the sky is the limit. Because when it's a complete passion you begin to evolve and realize, "I am working to enjoy my life." The same also goes for the rest of your life, especially your free time. Let's say you decide to set aside 2-3 hours per day just for you. How are you going to make that happen? Also, what are you going to do with those hours once you have them? The answer? Plan. Take apart your life in increments of 5, 10, even 15 minutes. How do they fit together? What do you do with those minutes? How can you begin to track these things? Where are the bottlenecks (eg. Where does business and family time meet and is there friction there?)?. Just like friction can kill your business machine, so can it kill a marriage or what was once a good life. Another example would be your retirement plan—if you have one. Get the picture? If not we'll cover this in a different way in a little while.

STEP 2 - COMMON MISTAKES YOU DON'T WANT TO MAKE

You'll always find it easy to stay where you are. Remember the old bromide: Don't rock the boat? I'm going to tell you that if you don't rock the boat you will NEVER achieve any more than you are currently achieving. WOW! You need to hear this over and over again. It's so important that you grasp this statement. I do not mean just read it, you need to believe it. Say it so many times to yourself that it becomes easier and easier for you to rock the boat, rather than sit in the boat! I know you want more than the status quo, because you're reading these words. Once you begin paying attention you'll find that everything in the universe is moving. Nothing is staying the same. Why would you think everything in your business can stay the same? You need to be on the constant lookout for things that seem out of the norm. These are areas that no one else is looking at. These are the very things that will propel you ahead of the pack!. Don't be fooled by the fact that it may seem outrageous! You need to understand that all of the best run businesses in the world also don't accept the norm! For example, they spend millions of dollars on surveys. Customer surveys, past customer surveys, employee surveys, supplier surveys, and there are many more. All these surveys keep the businesses from accepting the norm, it keeps and keep them digging below the surface of their businesses so that they are always listening to and watching the machine. Does it need an adjustment here? Maybe. How about over there? Definitely. It's not a coincidence that such companies are profitable. Why, then, would you accept the norm? You need to answer this honestly. It's the only way.

One of the most common mistakes a business can make is to not follow up. You must keep checking on your progress to profit. How will you know if you're there if you don't know where you are? Good written plans are essential. You will find that your financial institution will be impressed when you have one. Do you know the saying, "No one flies by the seat of their pants?" You shouldn't either. Action plans are difficult to do. Don't waste them, and don't be afraid to update them. These plans form the operational manual for your business and, as such, they're your success system.

Another mistake is not listening to others in your business. You're the master and creator of your company. You're the boss! You're busy doing all those things that need to get done. You hold the reins and you control the team. These are some of the reasons it makes it why it is difficult for you to hear what others are saying in your business. But know this: you need to be open and hear what others are saying. You need to be free to accept what's heard and then be brave to actually try what is proposed. You will find that, as you take the time to listen to your people, there's often merit in what's spoken. In the beginning you'll find that people are reluctant because you're the boss. It's uncomfortable for others to be telling you something that you may deem to be none of their "business." But that's the point, you see. A good employee treats your business as his or her own and wants to see it succeed as much as you do. So, you need to persevere, because when they do speak up, it will help you so much it will be hard to believe. This is one change that will move you forward in many ways.

No Branding ... You may think branding is something like a name or like a marking on something to signify ownership. This is somewhat true, but the correct answer definition is as follows. Branding is where you're special in the eyes of your customers. You're the top in your field in their eyes. You truly stand out above the crowd. You have the ability to do something that puts you above all your competitors. Your customers will think of you first, not second or third. You must be unique, and it doesn't just happen. You have to make it happen. You cannot say "I've been in business for a long time and therefore I've got a brand." That isn't how it works. You have to be doing something different from your competition down the street or down the road. They may have been in business for a long time also. You must find something that gives you a unique difference from others and then promote it to the fullest.

STEP 3 - BETTER TOOLS IN YOUR TOOLBOX

The following six items are some of the best tools in your toolbox, yet many small businesses such as yours never get the best value from them.

Pen and paper. Yes, pen and paper are the best tools a businessman can have. It is with these that you will draw up a business plan, which should be the central and the most important document you have. It can tell you at any given moment where your business is, as compared to where you want it to be. It has all your financials with respect to every single part of your business. It's your go-to guide to success.

So ... Forget what you've heard about jobs that can't be tied to revenue or that are considered "grin and bear it" costs of doing business. It just isn't true. A business is a machine that makes money. Every cog, screw and belt has a function, and each plays some role in the sales cycle as well as representing some form of expenditure. Teach your employees how each of your individual parts fits into your sales cycle and what the cost of each is to the company (in both acquisition and ongoing costs—like how many units must be sold to replace a damaged one), then expect everyone to take an active role in achieving company sales targets and budgets, reducing costs and promoting synergy.

Every employee should have sales-specific tasks. They should also be taught to focus on finding ways to reduce costs without affecting the quality of your service and products. And they should understand how each position within the company meshes with and supports all others. Why? All employees (and systems) receive a consistent portion of every dollar you earn. Increased synergy, higher sales and lower costs put more money into each of everyone's pockets. This is accomplished by constructing and following a business plan. Find an example plan online and begin your business plan now. And when you're done, look into constructing a marketing plan—another indispensable company document.

A Complete List of all the Services you Provide. Having a complete list of the services you and your employees provide—and having everyone in your employ memorize it—means that they'll always be at the tip of your tongues and ready to be spoken to a prospective customer. "Yes, we have a mechanic who does nothing but work on foreign cars. Your vehicle will be in good hands," says the service writer, rather than just taking the car in like any other. Now he has established your business in the mind of this customer as someplace he can bring his foreign car. Nice job of branding, there.

Two Years of Financial Statements. Why would you want two years of financial statements at your fingertips? Well, like the business plan and the marketing plan, these documents give you important current information as it's required. Let's say you want to stage a contest as to how many automatic starters your service people can sell in the second quarter of the year, the purpose being to obtain 10% growth over the same time last year (because the financial statements showed sales over the past two years were stagnant). If you keep detailed financial statements—and you really should—then you can quickly take last year's sales and use the figure to calculate what number of automatic starters sold will give you 10% growth. Split that number between your service people or your service person and yourself and you've got sales goals for each person to shoot for and maybe even beat. That's awesome!

Customer List. Your customer list is money in your pocket. It holds the contact information of everyone who's ever done business with you. Now let's say you're offering some kind of new service; a rust proofing outfit. Never was there a better time to send out a sales letter out to all of your customers, telling them what a great product it is, the benefits it will provide to their car, and that they can get the new service at a 10% discount for the first month it's available. Similarly, this list can be used to send Christmas cards or Birthday birthday cards (yes, you should always ask a customer when their birthday is). I subscribe to an online service that allows me to send any type of ecard from a wide selection of cards (yes, you should always ask for a customer's email). I also mail such cards to customers who still prefer regular mail. The rule of thumb is you should touch base three times per year with each of your customers—and not only when you wish to sell them something.

Competitors. Yes, you should have a list of competitors, what services and products they provide, what types of vehicles they work on, what kinds of equipment they have and don't have, and any single piece of information you can glean about them. Why? If the guy two blocks down the street has a great big sign saying he offers rust proofing, you might want to put up a sign saying you provide a certain type of battery or those car starters we talked about (because your list tells you he doesn't offer either of these products).

You don't want to go head to head with him. It just doesn't make sense. And let's say someone comes in ... you work on the car, do up the bill and then let them know that they really should be getting a front-end alignment done. They say okay, but you don't have the proper machine to do the job. That list of competitors will come in handy, as you'll be able to tell your customer where they can get the work done. He or she will remember this. And they'll keep coming back to you for other things.

Market Data. This one is a little more difficult, but important none-the-less. For example, it's not necessarily a good time to expand your business when the market is shrinking. That's a hard pill to swallow, but it's the best way to protect your business in that kind of a situation. Also, one doesn't want to have a large inventory going into what is typically your slow season. And do you even know which month? On average is your busiest of the year? Again, on average, what services and products are sold in that month? Do you have the raw materials on hand for quick service, or do your suppliers know this is going to be your busiest month? What can you prepare for? What can't you prepare for? How are you going to deal with these situations?

See what I'm getting at? As a business owner you should always keep on top of industry happenings (your market), both on a small and a large scale. Know your seasons well so that you can maximize both sales and service. And even pay attention to the marketplace at large. People tend to spend more when the markets are good than they do when the markets are bad. What campaigns can you run in either market to make the best use of your customer base?

STEP 4 - TAKE BABY STEPS

I've thrown a lot at you in a very short space of time. If the things I've been writing about are new to you, you're probably feeling overwhelmed. Take a deep breath! Let it out slow and relax. No goal of worth is easily reached, so your path must be approached in small, measured steps: baby steps! That's right. You're on a journey to a better place, and if you don't want to miss all the glorious sights along the way, you should break your long-term goal(s) into fun, short-term goals.

You know, it takes but a minute to change your behaviour and, thus, the results you get from life. The following daily recipe helps you put your focus on producing small, specific behaviours (and results) that move you toward the future you want. The reasoning is simple: If you consistently move toward a specific destination, you must eventually reach it. The following technique does just what we've been talking about:

1. Waking up: Start each day with questions designed to get you excited, enthusiastic and energized.

Example: What can I do, right now, that will make me feel excited, enthusiastic, and that will get me moving with the energy of a peak performer? If your mind replies that you should dance around the house like a maniac—do it!

2. Taking action: Action creates emotion. Anytime you feel yourself faltering, ask the question "What can I do, right now, that will allow me to enjoy myself and pursue my goals?" Do it! (I always refer to my prioritized list of goals when I ask this question.)

3. Creating focus: Target something you're thinking about, feeling, saying or doing at this moment. Is this behaviour moving you closer to your goals? If not, what thoughts, feelings, words or actions can you choose that will move you in the direction you want to go? Do these things!

Repeat step 3 on a regular basis throughout the day, especially when switching tasks, making decisions or choosing a course of action. It's also a great exercise when you find yourself getting drowsy.

4. Free time activities:

a) Still have lots of energy? Check your goal/priority lists for work, play, education and spiritual development—whatever: What task tops the list you selected? Do it!

b) Need to add to your list of things to do? Want to work on something different? Identify a problem related to your goals:

- What's the problem?
- What are all the possible solutions?
- What's the best one?
- How can you get from where you are now to the place where this solution has taken place? List these tasks and prioritize them.
- Do the first task on the list. Now!

c) Want to sit for a while? Brainstorm:

- Describe one of your current problems in a single sentence. Record this statement at the top of a blank sheet of paper.

- Write down everything you can think of that could help you solve the problem. No idea is too dumb.
- Keep at it for at least 15 minutes.
- Highlight the best ideas for future use.
- Better yet, start working at the best idea right now.

d) Feeling lethargic? Need some motivation? Develop some reasons for action: Using the brainstorming method just described, select some tasks you want to accomplish and list reasons for following through. Hint: People do things for only two reasons—to avoid pain or to gain pleasure.

5. Turning in:

- Before going to bed, make a list of tasks for tomorrow.
- Prioritize these goals, and make a promise to yourself to complete each in order of importance.
- Prepare your morning questions.

Put your focus on results, and never look away. You'll get to where you want to be. I know you will!

STEP 5 - BUILDING THE MACHINE

Before we get into building the machine, let's take a look at what it is we're going to construct. Here's a standard business model:

- Money, People & Product

- Generate Revenue
- Overhead, Marketing, Sales and Distribution
- Generate Expenses
- Revenue minus Expenses
- Generate Profit or Loss

To build the machine before us we need start-up money, at least one person, and a product to sell. (In this case product refers to both it and also refers to services.) These three things put together represent the minimum we need to start a business (Defined as an entity that Solves Problems and Generates Revenue). However, something happens when we begin to solve problems. We run into things that Generate Expenses. These are your Overhead Expenses (Everything from office space to buying a much needed tool); Marketing (The money spent to create a position in your prospective customer's head—something like, "Bob's is the place to go to get my Volkswagen fixed."); Sales (The money it costs you to make your sales); and Distribution (Costs experienced getting your Product to your Customer). Now we tally up everything that was spent to create Revenue and subtract the Expenses from Total Revenue. The difference is our Profit or Loss. What a rough way to start up a business! But believe me, it's done that way more often than you would think.

What, then, is the right way to build the machine? Use market information to build a solid business plan. It's only a detailed tool that lists every expected cost and all expected revenue and that can give you a document you can use as a daily, weekly and monthly guide to stay on track.

And you don't stop using the business plan when things begin to run smoothly. This is a living document that you'll use for the rest of your business days.

STEP 6 - SEVEN STEPS TO SUCCESS

Search: One must know what it is he or she is going to pursue. This may seem self-evident, but very few people know how to set goals. I'm talking about a statement of intention that is clear, to the point, is measurable and has a definite deadline. "I'm going to take an airplane flight to New York City on the 17th of July." As opposed to, "I'm thinking about taking a trip to New York this summer." Do you see the difference? The first statement can be broken down into smaller goals. The second statement can't be broken down as of yet. It isn't clear enough. It doesn't define the voyage we're contemplating. And the deadline is far too open-ended to be of much use.

Analyze: One must study the goal that has been set. Is it reasonable? Can it be broken down into ever smaller tasks until one arrives at a place or places where something can be done to begin the journey—today? Does the reverse engineered plan seem attainable to you?. If not, are there more steps that can be broken down into action steps? And so on ...

Determine: A list of tasks has been arrived at. One must discern which of these have merit. This is a further streamlining of the goal.

Choose: And finally, one must choose the first step, and the second, and so on. Because, in the end, all we have is choice. Yes or No; Good or Bad; Right or Wrong, Forward or Backward; Up and Down, etc.

Action: But a choice is not the beginning of a journey. A journey suggests motion. And that's where action comes in. Many small movements (baby steps) can lead to massive action over time.

Measurement: One must ascertain whether or not a set of actions (goals) is moving the individual closer to his destination. Has the journey been pleasant (as planned for)? Have the tiny steps been keeping you on course? And this is the most important question: are you still on course? Because if you aren't, one must begin again with a search for the proper action to correct the course. Just as a ship on the sea modifies its direction time and again to stay on target, so must you.

Change: If the measurement shows you have gotten off course, then you must make the suggested change in direction. I know everyone hates change, but the successful businessperson must embrace change; it's the only way he or she will make it through the maze that is the life of a business.

STEP 7 - PERSEVERANCE IS KEY

Perseverance is the key to a successful business. You must be able to continually deal with problems (after all that's what business is: the solving of problems for your customers). This ability is dependent on a number of things: the belief that you can do what lies before you, the ability to make the right choices at the right time, and the inner strength to act on those choices over and over again, just to mention a few. The following list is meant to help you maintain your momentum, to persevere when you're finding it hard to keep making and acting on the right choices.

First of all, don't try moving mountains. When faced with monumental issues learn to go around them, over them, under them or even through them, because if you try to move the entire mountain it will always outlast you;, it may even break you. It's much like the idea of being able to bend with the wind without breaking. Some problems are insurmountable and one can't stop the wind. So you must learn to make different choices, to access different beliefs and to lean on that inner strength I know you have.

Confidence: Be confident in your ability to make moment to moment choices that will help keep your momentum. Remember that everything comes down to a single choice: yes or no, etc. and that you have the ability to make that choice. If you don't choose to say yes or no, aren't you making a decision not to respond to the question or problem before you? That's like putting a blindfold on and saying "I'm going to pretend the mountain isn't there." That will almost guarantee a crash, don't you agree?

Get help: In situations where you're momentum is in danger, another option is asking for help. Don't be afraid to go to your employees and ask them to help deal with the problem before you. You can also look to a mentor or a friend—someone you can bounce ideas off or who may even have the experience necessary to offer you a solution. Being the boss is a lonely place to be at times, make sure you don't isolate yourself any more than you already have. If the stress remains, why not consider talking to a professional? Social services counselors, psychologists and psychiatrists can offer you skills for coping with and solving problems.

Rewards: There are very few tools that are as powerful, with respect to perseverance, than giving yourself (and your employees) rewards. I always reward myself and others for jobs well done or for working through a particularly difficult problem. These don't have to be spectacular awards. A couple of tickets to the movies for an employee (and his spouse) for as a thank you for dealing with a particularly difficult customer will motivate beyond your wildest expectations. Treating yourself to a nice dinner as a reward for coming in on budget this month will help you to prepare for next month. An ice cream cone for a particularly good day marks the occasion in your mind and leaves you more prepared for tomorrow's problems. Take my word for it, rewards work.

Erase self-doubt: "I'm unsure" is one of the greatest signs of procrastination. You're always better off choosing action over inaction. Even if it proves to be one of your poorer decisions, sitting on the fence post is no place for a business person to be. That's like stopping before the proverbial mountain and waiting for erosion to wear it down. It's just bad thinking. Better to ask a question like, "What's the best choice that is available to me at the moment?" and then picking one of the answers that appear in your mind. (Your mind will always give you answers. That's its job. All you have to do is ask.)

One of the greatest fears a businessperson faces is losing customers. The next one is the fear of losing the business. If you establish the business model and business plan laid out for you earlier, you'll know almost immediately if you're losing business, and it will also give you a check list you can go to in order to begin figuring out where, exactly, your machine is breaking down. And you'll never have to worry about losing your business if you pay close attention to your business plan. It will tell you where problems are long before they ever become business killers. The only way you'll ever be in danger is if you fail to respond to business problems as they occur. This is what kills most businesses. Don't be one of them.

80-20 Rule: It's amazing how many areas of business and life fall under the shadow of the 80:20 rule. Want a successful business? Understand that 20% of your customers will give you 80% of your business. Does this mean you ignore the other 80% of customers? Absolutely not! You never know when a small fish will become a big fish. You also want to be known as a terrific businessperson, a place to send your friends to. This means that everyone must get great service. The top 20%? Well, you'll just have to pull out all the stops and also come up with the best rewards you can think of to give them for their patronage. Everyone enjoys being made to feel special. You can do this!

Do you know where most of your business problems will come from? 80% of your problems will arise from 20% of your customers. It's alright to fire some of these people. That's right: if you can't win over a difficult customer, don't spend a lot of time worrying about it. Just let him or her go. Send them to another shop. Let them have the headache!

80% of the rest of your problems will be financial and will fall into one of four areas. Look at your business model. It's laid out for you. Overhead, Marketing, Sales, and Distribution. You say you want to double your profits? Here's how you do it in one fell swoop: become a great accountant, an expert marketer, a super salesperson and a magician of a distributor. The better you are in these areas the better will be your business and your profits. And if you don't have the time or the inclination to do these things? I have two answers for you:

1. Hire top people, particularly an accountant, a marketing manager, a sales manager and a distribution manager.

2. Get out of business. I'm not joking about this. The four areas mentioned will take or should take up to 100% of your business expenses.

Here's the breakdown of projected business expenses for most any successful business: Overhead 20%, Marketing 20%, Sales 20%, Distribution 20%, PROFIT 20%. I'm sure you can manage your overhead expenses, but are you a great marketing person, great salesperson and a great distributor? Most business people are not experts in all these areas. You must make the choices as to how to solve these problems. Make them soon, please.

Visit my website for more information and examples:
www.profitfortheautomotiveserviceindustry.com

How to Make Your Advertisement Infinitely More Effective

FRANCIS ABLOLA

What we're going to talk about in this chapter is how to focus a laser beam on your target audience when advertising. It's not going to be about writing your sales letter and writing your copy. I'm a direct response copywriter. What that means is I write copy that produces results immediately. But before any single word is written on a page, I want to make sure that I have the audience in mind. How do I do this? Through mind reading. I know it's a little funny to talk about mind reading, but How to Make Your Advertisement Infinitely More Effective is really about getting inside the customer's mind and figuring out exactly what that individual desires. There's a quote I want to share with you. It's by Robert Collier, who's one of the greatest copywriters to ever live. It states, "Always enter the conversation already taking place in the customer's mind."

Now if you're not taking notes right now, you should be. I want you to write this down ... "Always enter the conversation already taking place in the customer's mind." Because as we go through each day, all of us have something that's so pressing in our heads that we need to just get it out into the world. If someone can actually go in there, into our heads, and solve the problem for us, the one that we're thinking about constantly, it immediately cuts through the clutter of everyday thinking and allows them to really reach us. So, that's what we're going to talk about, how you can get into the customer's mind with your marketing.

My promise for everybody reading this is that I'm going to walk you through some powerful influence strategies for increasing the effectiveness of any marketing, of any business or any stage of business. If you're just getting started, you need to know this information; if you've been in business for years, if you're a veteran, and you're not doing this in your business right now, you're leaving money on the table because your advertising is not as effective as it could be.

Did you ever wish that you were a super hero? I think we all might have at some time in our lives. And as a marketer there's one super power that I would want and that's the ability to read people's minds. I would want to get into their heads and actually figure out what they want, even if they, themselves, don't truly know what they want. That's really what we're going to talk about today. It's marketing mind reading.

Now imagine having the power to focus only on attracting your ideal customers, having the ability to build trust instantly with everyone you work with, being able to stay on top of the mind of someone who's looking at your advertising, someone who could be a potential customer of yours, with the power to channel existing wants and desires into your business.

Let's say your business already channels the existing wants and desires of your customers. Can you imagine having the power to press all their emotional hot buttons and psychological triggers so that you send them into a buying frenzy? Wouldn't you like that?

Businesspeople—they have a product, it's their baby. They like to think they know everything that everybody wants, but it's simply not the truth. Yet, that's what we're going to go into today. Imagine having a magical marketing crystal ball that tells you exactly how your ideal customer is thinking and feeling. Now we all can't have that magic ball, but you can use top secret intelligence to create irresistible advertising that fuels your business.

I'm super excited to share that top secret intelligence with you today. When you do these things, you make your ideal customers pay attention. Now, we're so bombarded with information, it's hard to focus on anything. But if you really make your ideal customers pay attention to you, that's a very, very strong thing you can do. They should see you as a trusted advisor and a friend and an authority. Being an authority in your marketplace is a must. Being able to turn that authority into more leads, more loyal customers and eventually more sales, well that's the ultimate super power.

I think everybody reading this wants more sales, so I hope you're with me on that. It really doesn't matter if you're just getting started, if you've been in business for decades or what nature of industry you're in. A lot of people say, "Well, my business is different." Using this strategy, this thing I'm about to show you, every business is the same—because human nature is the same. And that's really what we're planning on using in our advertising.

What I want to show you today is going to help you make an immediate, dramatic impact to your product. But before we go on, I want to answer the question: who the heck is this guy? Some of my early mentors were Les Brown, the legendary Jim Rohn (who was the mentor of Tony Robbins) and William Bailey (who was the mentor Les Brown and Jim Rohn). Today, I'm considered a top marketing and advertising strategist. I work with Fortune 1000 companies, and I've also worked with garage start-ups. Lots of multimillion-dollar CEOs, and New York Times best-selling authors. I've been featured in papers and websites all around the country. I'm also the number-one Amazon best selling author of The Art and Science of Success, with many other best-selling authors. The gurus actually call on me to produce more revenue for their advertising campaigns. This strategy that I'm sharing with you, is going to help you do the same. I've helped my clients create millions in revenue, hundreds of thousands of new leads and customers in rapid speed.

But none of that stuff really matters. What really matters is getting what's inside of my head working for you as if you had a mini me helping grow your business. Let's really get started, because everything we're going to show is actionable, and immediately beneficial to you.

Here's the big problem: we're all overloaded with information. We're overloaded, you're overloaded, your prospects and your customers are overloaded. It's been said that we are bombarded with some 3000 advertisements per day. How do we get our prospect's attention? That's really what we're fighting for with everything going on in the world today. The first solution that everyone goes to is advertise. But how do we know we're doing the right thing? There are so many things we can do … TV, radio, internet, social media, press releases and online classified ads. There are so many different channels as a marketer, and as an advertiser, that we can use. But how do we know it's effective? How do we know we're using our time the right way? How do we know we're using our money the right way? As an entrepreneur, I'm sure you'd agree that money and time are the two most important things in a business.

So really what we want to do is focus in on effective advertising. And here's what effective advertising does ... Effective advertising focuses on the right media to the right potential customer. If your advertising doesn't do that, if it goes to a broad audience, you may be losing money. Does your advertisement speak directly to your target audience? Effective advertising speaks to the person who's reading it. Not only that, but it is benefit driven to what your ideal customer wants. Not what the marketer wants but what they're customer is looking for. And finally, it has a specific call-to-action. If you're advertising doesn't do this, you may be leaving money on the table.

As an example, you wouldn't stick a realtor sign up on the front lawn of a home to attract a million-dollar buyer, would you? Really, it's comparing your advertising to a shotgun, versus a sniper rifle. All of your advertising should be the sniper rifle, especially if you have a small budget to work with.

Here's the bad news: all of your customers are ignoring you. You really need to cut through the clutter. You need to get their attention with laser focus and that sniper rifle approach. So, who do your customers listen to? I've eluded to this earlier, they listen to trusted friends and advisors. They listen to people who understand their needs, their problems and have their best interest in mind. David Ogilvy, one of my legendary heroes in marketing, wrote, "All good marketing requires empathy." It's very important, it's another writer-downer, if you're taking notes. "All good marketing requires empathy." That means having a connection with your target audience but calling them a person, because that's what they really are.

So how do you reach all these real people? Too many business owners tend to get their advertising and their marketing done the wrong way. One of the ways they get marketing done wrong is they try to sell the features and not the benefits of what someone is looking for. They market to what they think is important verses what the customer's looking for. They don't think what the customer thinks is important.

Now, there may be some people out there thinking, "Well, that's not me. I didn't do this when I started my marketing campaigns, and we're making a lot of good money right now." But the fact is, it doesn't matter if you're losing money or making money, if you don't know your customer market—even if you're doing well with your marketing—chances are you can probably increase your sales and conversions. It doesn't always mean you're going to fail by not using this approach first, but it almost always means you're going to increase conversions by going back and doing this kind of research.

Here's what I want to stress today. You can be a terrible advertisement copywriter, but as long as you know your market with pinpoint accuracy, you can create effective advertising. My advice might seem counter-intuitive ... and that's to stop selling to customers. Instead, you want to listen to your customers, and you want to become their best friends, their BFFs. The reason why is because you want to position yourself as a trusted advisor offering valuable guidance to your best friend. That puts you in a completely different category from all the people who aren't listening to your market but are just trying to sell to them.

When you become a trusted advisor, you become the first person this customer listens to. You become their expert and their authority. You become your target market--thinking what they think, feeling what they feel, going where they go, and experiencing what they experience.

Now, I became a really good copywriter in my niche, but not because I'm a great writer. In fact, I barely made it out of college English. I barely made it out of high school. The reason I became a really good copywriter in my niche is because I understand what my audience is looking for. I actually go to seminars as an attendee to talk with the people who are there, to do my market research, to get into their heads, to feel what they feel and to experience what they experience.

If you're selling to a market, and it's your primary market, you want to become that market, not a person selling to them. This is so vitally important. Stop thinking customer, prospect, or name on a list. Start thinking "real person" with hopes, dreams, wants, needs, desires, and problems only you can solve.

I have a funny approach to doing this that I call making up "imaginary best friends" for fun and profit. Because I love my best friends. And becoming someone's best friend is the next best thing to climbing into their head and reading their mind. Again, going back to the super powers that we all wish we had, mine is being able to read somebody's mind. If you can't read somebody's mind, the next best thing is becoming best friends with them, because best friends tell each other secrets. They tell each other hopes and dreams and desires. They let you know what they want, why they want it, what they like, who they trust, why they trust them, and why they buy.

If I consider you a really good friend, we share things that we wouldn't share to the general public. And I'm sure people reading this today have the same thing with their best friend. So, I want you to imagine being best friends with your marketplace. And here's the thing, your imaginary best friends? What we do is call it creating customer personas, or often times creating customer avatars. Basically, it's a clear, written profile of specific segments of your target audience.

When you have this, you can actually identify to the "T" who the person your ideal customer is. You want to focus on attracting who will give you the most money with the least resistance. This may seem like I'm saying you should get more for doing less. But it's not; it's about making the most money with the least amount of resistance.

Zero in on your best customers. Zero in on the people who you enjoy working with, and who also enjoy working with you. Think about it ... Would you rather work with the guy who enjoys going golfing a couple of afternoons per week, or another guy, the party animal? The answer really depends on what you want and what you have to offer. But the marketing is different, the advertising is different, to go after these two different groups of people. When you're creating imaginary friends, it really helps to interact with your target customer on a deeper, individual basis. After all, what you're doing here is building a lifestyle business.

You always want to think in terms of what benefits they want, not what you can offer them; not what you think they want, but what they're actually looking for. You must remember this for when you get into the marketplace, for when you create these imaginary friends, for when you truly begin to understand what they're looking for, because you might come to find out they're looking for something completely different than what you have to offer and that they're only working with you because that's the closest thing. This is exciting, because you now have the opportunity to get more money or work from them by creating a different relationship—all because they're looking for something that's not on the market. Who knows? This could even be a new opportunity for you and your business.

Creating imaginary friends also guides your marketing: it guides your brand, it guides design, and it guides advertising messages that speak to the proper audience. Again, we're seeing the shotgun versus the sniper rifle approach. So let's make some imaginary friends. I'm about to walk you through a process that I use whenever I create a marketing piece for a new audience, or a new market.

I'd like to say I'm not alone, because I have my imaginary friends who are helping me write my marketing. Again, this is the guide to effective advertising, even before writing a single word on a page, or creating a single ad. It's creating these imaginary friends, who tell you exactly what your market's looking for.

STEP 1

The first step is to brainstorm. It's sitting down with a pad and paper and just thinking. "Who are your best customers? Who are they currently? What type of customers do you want to attract? Who would you consider a best customer for you?" When you create these imaginary friends, think of them as they fit into each segment of your customer base. You don't need only one imaginary best friend, you can have multiple imaginary friends who all speak to a different audience.

You want to give them names and personalities, even jobs and families. Be very specific with the information you already know. If you already have customers, you can say, "Well, this is Bob. Bob works full-time, but he also works on the side as a real estate investor. He's looking to be more effective. You know, Bob works 40 hours a week in his regular job, and he spends about 20 hours a week in his real estate investing business. He also has a family and two kids that he tries to juggle with, and he's very frustrated with the results he's getting in this side business."

Knowing all this information, you get to know Bob a little bit better, and how to help him even more. So far this is really just an educated guess, because the next thing you want to do is actually go out in market and prove it. You want to go gather the data. You want to see, do these people really exist? The best way to do that is to actually go and look to your existing customers, go and talk to them. Talk to anybody in your company who interacts with your customers on a daily basis. If you have sales people in your company, for example, talk to them. Maybe talk to them about their best customers.

If you have a best customer in mind, talk to them, ask them what they want. Start doing interviews. The best thing you can do, the easiest thing, is you can survey your list by using a tool like SurveyMonkey or Wufoo. These let you create free forms to send out via email, asking your list of "friends" questions that will help you get to know them better. And by getting to know them better, your advertising becomes much more effective, because you gear all of your marketing message directly to these friends. This is actually how I won the award for copywriter of the year and became the guru's go-to guy. In my market I write heavily to people who want to learn how to become real estate investors. So I go where they go, and I get to know them. I actually go to seminars and sit in the back of the room. I talk to people who are attending—just like I was the seminar for the first time.

I get to know them better, and I find ways to understand them better, to feel what they feel, to understand their emotions, to experience the experiences they go through. And by doing that you discover so many things about your target market that you'll never know just from graphs and data and not seeing customers face-to-face. It's super important to do this, to get to know them and become friends with them. Open up a conversation (and it's amazing to know what kinds of information people give just by opening up a conversation).

STEP 2

The next step is to dig deeper. From the information you've gathered, from the brainstorming you've done and from all the proof you've backed it up with, you want to ... understand who they are, what they want, how they buy, why they buy, and what would get them to buy from you? Obviously, this is a very important question.

STEP 3

Now is the time to create your customer profile. That's right: create a profile of your imaginary friends, and make them as real as possible. I even go to the extent of finding a picture that best represents the person. I actually go to Google images or use a service like iStockphoto or Dreamstime. If you know your target market is male, in his 40s or 50s, with a family, you can actually go to istockphoto.com and find photos of people just like that.

By having these profiles and by getting them as real as possible, you can create this avatar, this persona, this imaginary friend who you can speak to and write to. Just the other day, we were talking to one of my copywriter friends on an interview we did, and he was referencing another copywriter who's a very successful copywriter. On her first promotion she was writing to a market her mother actually fit into. So as her customer avatar, as her persona, and as her imaginary friend, she actually set a picture of her mom in front of her laptop, and as she wrote the letter and the advertising piece, she wrote it as if she was writing to her mother. The advertisement piece was a well-liked hit, and it was very, very successful. Imagine you're writing your advertising to someone you truly care about, who you truly want to see a difference in. This is when and why your advertising becomes so much more powerful.

Here's what you want to ask when you're really digging into creating these imaginary friends. The first one is demographics, it's the who they are. Let's say this is Bob. What do we want to know about Bob? We want to know where he lives, his age group, marital status, occupation, job status and income. Does he own a home, does he rent? What's his education and reading level? That's really important, especially when you're creating an advertisement. What kind of lifestyle does he live? What kind of things interest him? What are his special interests? Maybe it's political interest, something like that. And political affiliations are very important to know, because obviously political affiliations really drive a person's character and how they operate. For example, you don't want to write a message that has a Democrat overtone to a Republican audience. It doesn't work that way.

STEP 4

The next thing is psychographics. This is about what they want and how they see themselves. What's their personal attitude toward themselves? Are they confident or are they not confident about their future? How do you use that in your advertising? How do they interact with you and other people? What are their personality types? Are they outgoing or are they soft-spoken? It's really important to know how to approach a target audience through their certain mannerisms. What are their beliefs? Again, really important. You want to make sure that you're not offending your target audience, but you also don't want to go too soft and make them ignore your advertising. What kind of affiliations in other groups do they have? What's their social status? Where do they see themselves in the world, and how the world reacts to them? What kind of books do they enjoy reading? This is really important. You're getting back into the conversation that's going in their head. If you know they're a huge Twilight fan (Twilight was a huge book on the market), you could actually use Twilight in your advertisement—maybe as a subject line? What websites have they visited? Also note that they're diehard Huffington Post readers. Why? If you've created an advertisement that actually talked about the Huffington Post it would attract them and actually get them to open the advertisement. What kind of hobbies do they do? Again, if they have strong beliefs in a certain hobby, how do you use that in your marketing? And what drives them on a day-to-day basis? Note: All these questions are important, but I think more important than the demographic information, is what they want and how they interact with you.

I also want to add a quick word about websites. I love forums. I love forums because people go to forums to talk with somebody in the same exact niche. It's two people having a conversation who are friends. Everybody chimes in, so you get to know your market well. Dashboards.com is a great website for finding niche forums like that. People open up and act like themselves inside of forums because they're not buying stuff. They feel like they can talk like they would normally talk to their friends. A point to add to the forums is that when people interact on forums, they're actually hidden by their usernames. They can even share their deepest feelings. This goes back to getting into where your market goes. It's not even real life, person-to-person, but it's going to allow you to see them where they spend time and interact with others. Very important, I love this strategy.

Going back to the point of what drives them on a day-to-day basis, what do they focus on? Are they focusing on just surviving a daily life? Or are they looking to connect with others? Are they looking for affluence and significance in their family life? Are they looking for enjoyment on a daily basis? When you understand the true psychological need, what they need to fulfill, your advertising becomes much more effective.

STEP 5

Find the pain. What's really eating away at them, day and night? What's the primary need your imaginary friend is desperate to fill? What's the biggest problem that's always on their mind? What keeps them up at night? Get into the conversation that's already happening on an everyday basis. What problems are they trying to solve in their lives? What's the biggest benefit they want? When you start thinking of what needs they are desperate to fill, and approaching your marketing that way, it becomes so much more effective because it clears the clutter. It stops you from saying "Here's what I think is important to you," but, rather, allows you to say, "This is what seems to be important from your point of view." You begin to be able to understand what influences their decisions. Again, this is a very important part of understanding who your customer is and what is their ultimate goal in buying from or interacting with you. Why are they looking to buy this product or service, if they don't know that they want to buy this product or service? What needs are they looking to fill that will get them to respond to your advertising? What emotions do you want them to feel? Is it security, is it confidence? Do you want them to feel significant when they work with you or buy your product or service? Do you want to give them independence? Are they looking for independence when they buy or interact with you? Also is it fun for them? What would make it fun to work with you? Again, a very important thing to know. Do they trust you? Hopefully the message that has woven its way throughout this entire presentation will lead you to understand that the whole point is getting your customers to trust you as an advisor they can call upon and lean on. And finally, if they don't trust you yet, what has to happen for them to trust you? What are they looking for as a symbol of trust?

A good example of that last point is your mailbox. How many things do you get in the mail for free? People who are sending you free gifts are putting you in a "wow" state of mind, like, "This guy's great. He just gave me something free." It automatically breaks down barriers. But it's also building value upfront, so you have their trust later. This is very, very important. How do you stand out? How do you create that "wow" experience? How are you different? And how do you create that trust to carry you into a deeper relationship. When you're creating that trust, you want to create your trust with your ideal client, which takes us into what we we're going to talk about now, which is how do you focus only on your imaginary friend, who you can help and, more importantly, who wants your help? You can't help everyone, especially if they don't want to hear from you.

So how do you only work with those people who are actively looking for what you have to offer? How do you invest your time and energy on clients and customers who can help expand your business and move in the direction that you want? The answer? You only focus on working with clients and consumers who want that same thing you are offering and who will also support your lifestyle in terms of that.

You also want to avoid time wasters. Don't work with energy vampires, because these people will take your business away from you. Only focus on the imaginary friends, the customer group that most wants your help, and that you can help the most by giving them massive transformational value.

STEP 6

Put your imaginary friends to work. Now that you've created all these profiles, that you've put these pieces together, how do you put them to work?

The simplest thing is, think of your new imaginary friend every time you plan a new campaign, or craft, or sales message. Again, all of your advertising is driven (laser-focused) to that specific person. So as you're creating your marketing, as you're creating your websites and as you're creating your copy, think of, "Does my imaginary friend, or will my imaginary friend, respond to this piece of advertising?"

The next thing is to speak to that individual. Here's a trick: all of your advertisements should speak to an individual person, not a group. Because when we read advertisements, we don't feel like we're a group, we feel like we're a single person, because we really are. And your advertisements should portray that. Develop a relationship with your imaginary friend. The more you get to know your imaginary friends, the more you get to know your marketplace. The more you get to know your marketplace, the easier it is to speak to them through all of the advertisements you put out.

HERE ARE MY BIGGEST TAKEAWAYS

One, become your audience. Watch what they watch, read what they read, go where they go. Two, get into the mind of your ideal prospect. Enter the conversation. Three, focus your advertising on your market. Focus the benefit-driven message that your customer wants. Not you but what your customer wants. Four, the biggest takeaway is talk to your imaginary friend—because best friends share secrets.

I think that's all I've got. I hope you were taking notes, because the most important part of your business is finding out what your customers actually want. It doesn't matter whether you're doing terrible in your marketing efforts or if you think you're doing well, applying these techniques will skyrocket your conversions.

www.ingramcontent.com/pod-product-compliance
Lightning Source LLC
Chambersburg PA
CBHW072242270326
41930CB00010B/2239
* 9 7 8 1 7 7 2 7 7 1 4 9 7 *